Treating Common Diseases

Hugh McGavock BSc, MD, FRCGP

Visiting Professor of Prescribing Science
Department of Nursing Studies
University of Ulster
Course Organiser, GP Continuing Clinical Education
Northern Ireland Medical and Dental Training Agency

and

Dennis Johnston DSc, MD, PhD, FRCP, FRCPI

Whitla Professor of Therapeutics and Pharmacology
Queen's University Belfast
Consultant Physician, Belfast City Hospital

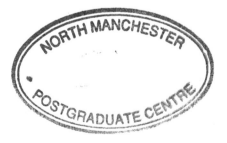

Radcliffe Publishing
Oxford • New York

Radcliffe Publishing Ltd
18 Marcham Road
Abingdon
Oxon OX14 1AA
United Kingdom

www.radcliffe-oxford.com
Electronic catalogue and worldwide online ordering facility

British Library Cataloguing in Publication Data

A catalogue record for this book is available from the British Library.

ISBN-13: 978 1 84619 183 1

Typeset by Anne Joshua & Associates, Oxford
Printed and bound by TJI Digital, Padstow, Cornwall

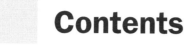

Contents

Preface

The study of disease and its treatment is a lifelong intellectual journey which has engaged some of humankind's finest minds and kindest hearts. We, the authors, are still on that fascinating voyage. Every journey begins with a single step, and that step is the purpose of this introductory book. It is short enough to be read from cover to cover, re-read, studied and learned. Those who do this should find that they understand much that they encounter in patients, whether in the wards, outpatient departments or in primary care.

Treating Common Diseases should also ease the student clinician's passage to more comprehensive texts, which can be intimidating in their volume and complexity if there has been no prior introduction.

Although this book is intentionally short, we have taken every care to ensure that it is as correct as modern research evidence can make it. Since most modern disease management involves the use of medicinal drugs, students may find it helpful to read the Radcliffe companion volume, *How Drugs Work* (second edition, published in 2005). This will help them to make the vital link between drug science (pharmacology) and drug treatment (therapeutics). The *British National Formulary* (*BNF*) is an essential companion for all clinicians, whether students or consultants!

The authors seek your comments on the book, whether positive or negative – the best critics are surely the readers! Welcome to the first step on your journey into therapeutics.

Hugh McGavock
Dennis Johnston
September 2007

Acknowledgements

Writing a short introductory clinical text is challenging, presenting many problems and potential pitfalls. Hugh McGavock is greatly indebted to the following clinical teachers, all medical specialists, for devoting time and expertise to reviewing his chapters: Dr Colin Kenny (Diabetes), Professor Stuart Elborn (Respiratory Disease), Dr Peter Watson (Gastroenterology), Dr Allister Taggart (Rheumatology), Dr Graeme McDonald and Dr Elizabeth McGavock (Psychiatry) and Dr Hugh Webb (Infectious Disease). We also wish to record our thanks to the staff of Radcliffe Publishing for their enthusiasm, expertise and courtesy.

To our wives, families, colleagues and students

Introduction

Selecting safe and effective treatment of diseases is a complex and intellectually demanding element of clinical practice. Faced with a range of treatments for a particular disease, it is often difficult to optimize, and optimal treatment may be missed. When an optimal regime is selected, the results are usually beneficial to the patient, making the most of the splendid advances in modern drug discovery and development. A suboptimal regime may worsen the patient's condition, sometimes leading to hospitalization and even death.

The scientific prescriber routinely makes the intellectual link between the science of pharmacology (how drugs work) and its application in disease management (therapeutics). The purpose of this book is to help you to train yourself to make that link at stage 1 of your career, and to go on making it at whatever level you practise. It is not so very difficult to achieve this, but it requires the mindset into which this book will encourage you:

- Am I sure of the diagnosis?
- Do I understand clearly what I am planning to do?
- Do I know which biological mechanisms I am targeting?
- Will my proposed treatment 'dovetail' safely with existing medication?
- Have I educated and convinced the patient (the senior partner in the therapeutic process) about what is proposed, mentioning the need for regular dosing?

However long you practise, and however senior you become, if you fail to 'scan' these questions before prescribing, you will not practise as effectively and safely as you ought.

The starting point

It is essential to have learned thoroughly the basic science of pharmacology, to which the Radcliffe text *How Drugs Work* is an introduction. Without at least that level of understanding, your prescribing will be akin to that of a cook using a well-tried recipe book! As *How Drugs Work* explains, most of the drugs that are prescribed for serious, long-term diseases, like raised blood pressure (hypertension) or diabetes, act at one of four biological 'targets' – the chemical signalling processes of the body cells. These are:

- receptors on the cell membrane or nucleus
- enzyme processes within or outside the cell
- ion channels in the cell membrane
- carrier (transporting) molecules in the cell membrane.

For some diseases, the prescriber may have the option of modifying all four of these 'targets', e.g. hypertension, and for others only two can be modified, e.g. asthma. If the decisions of good prescribing are in some ways like fitting together the pieces of a jigsaw puzzle, these four bio-targets are the pieces at the centre of the jigsaw.

Several other essential factors must also be taken into account in every prescribing decision:

- Are the patient's kidney and liver function normal? If not, the patient may be unable to process and excrete drugs adequately, and smaller doses than normal may be advisable.
- Is the patient elderly or very young? Both age groups 'handle' drugs differently from the general population aged 12–70 years.
- Is there a possibility of serious interaction between drugs (a) at their sites of action, (b) during their metabolism (inactivation) or (c) during their excretion? You must consider this possibility, using special computer software if necessary, both for your own prescription of two or more drugs and whenever adding to pre-existing drug treatment.
- What is the likelihood of unwanted effects from your treatment, on cells and organs other than the diseased ones? Many tissues share the same

chemical signalling processes which are essential for normal functioning of healthy organs. Modern drugs often block or stimulate these physiological signals and can consequently disrupt healthy organ function even as they improve the function of the diseased organ. This is a simple explanation of many unwanted side-effects of modern drugs. Benefit must always be balanced against risk, and *How Drugs Work* introduces you to all of these points.

- Is there coexisting disease? This may have a vital bearing on drug selection, further complicating your planning of optimal treatment.

- Can I persuade this patient to take the medicines well enough to achieve benefit – the right dose, at the right frequency, for the right length of time? Patients who fail to take their medicines properly fail to get the potential benefits. If your treatment fails, it is often due to non-compliance in one of several forms, and every prescriber must foster an informed therapeutic trust with each patient, particularly those on long-term maintenance therapy. Clinical science is powerless if the patient does not fulfil his or her part of the 'therapeutic contract.'

This short book explores the treatment options for some of the common major diseases of 'Western' society, and considers how to select scientifically the best current drug therapy for a particular patient. It is short enough to be studied from cover to cover and to be committed to memory, as a foundation on which to build your understanding of drug treatment, which can be adapted as newer drugs and knowledge appear.

Please note that drugs are referred to by their approved (generic) names, in keeping with best practice. Students may be confused by the frequent use of brand names in both hospital and primary care. The *British National Formulary* (*BNF*) will tell you what the brand name actually is, and which drug group it is a member of. Keep a *BNF* in your pocket!

1 Hypertension

Hypertension is the level of blood pressure above which treatment does more good than harm.

(Rose, 1980)

Blood pressure = cardiac output × total peripheral resistance.

Two factors contribute to the level of blood pressure, namely the cardiac output and the arterial resistance. In hypertensive patients, cardiac output is usually normal or slightly reduced whereas peripheral resistance is always increased. Therefore all currently available antihypertensive drugs lower blood pressure by dilating resistance vessels and reducing peripheral resistance. High-dose diuretics and beta-blockers can reduce cardiac output, but this does not represent their principal mode of action. In the early stages of hypertension, increased peripheral resistance is due to increased vascular tone and can be fully reversed by vasodilator therapy. In more established disease a combination of medial hypertrophy, reduced numbers of resistance vessels and impaired compliance in larger vessels leads to elevated blood pressure which is more difficult to control.

The diagnosis of hypertension is based on the clinic blood pressure. In adults (> 18 years) it is defined as a systolic blood pressure > 140 mmHg and/or a diastolic blood pressure > 90 mmHg. Measurements must be made under standardized conditions using accurate, validated and well-maintained devices with the appropriate cuff size. The level of blood pressure should be viewed in the context of overall cardiovascular risk. For primary prevention, assessment of risk can be defined using the risk tables at the back of the *British*

National Formulary. These help to define the need for therapy in mild hypertension and whether other interventions, particularly lipid-lowering therapy and aspirin, are indicated.

Measurement of blood pressure in the seated position after 10 minutes' rest is the recommended measurement, but standing blood pressure is necessary in elderly or diabetic patients to exclude orthostatic hypotension (a sudden fall in blood pressure on standing up, causing dizziness). In mild uncomplicated hypertension at least four pairs of measurements should be made over a period of 3–6 months before drug treatment is introduced. For those with established cardiovascular disease, target organ damage (damage to the heart, arteries, brain, retinae and kidneys, caused by prolonged hypertension) or severe hypertension, drug treatment should be initiated within weeks rather than months of observation.

Aims of treatment

The purpose of lowering blood pressure, especially when combined with lipid-lowering therapy and aspirin, is to prevent the development of cardiovascular disease. Patients rarely feel better when they receive anti-hypertensive therapy, although most first-line antihypertensive agents are well tolerated. For the majority, a target blood pressure of < 140/85 mmHg is recommended, but in patients with diabetes, chronic renal failure or established evidence of atherosclerosis, a target pressure of < 130/80 mmHg should be achieved.

Management

There is convincing evidence that weight reduction, moderate salt restriction and alcohol reduction lower blood pressure at least in the short term, and should be recommended. The health benefits of increased exercise, stopping smoking, and a diet rich in fruit, vegetables and fish oils are also convincing. At best, however, multiple lifestyle interventions result in reductions in blood pressure equivalent to drug monotherapy (treatment with a single drug) and should not be used as an alternative to drug therapy in patients whose blood pressure remains persistently elevated. Patients on drug treatment will also benefit from lifestyle interventions, especially salt restriction.

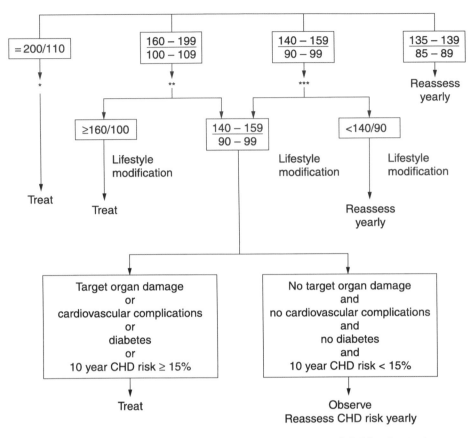

Figure 1.1: Diagnosis and management of hypertension.

Selection of drug therapy

Evidence from major cardiovascular outcome trials has consistently concluded that a decrease in blood pressure is the main factor in reducing morbidity and mortality. Beta-blockers are less effective in reducing events in older patients, and the combination with diuretics increases the risk of developing type 2 diabetes more than other drug combinations. Alpha-blockers are less effective than diuretics in preventing stroke and heart failure, and should now be considered third-line agents. For stroke prevention and in the elderly, thiazide diuretics, calcium-channel blockers and angiotensin-II-receptor antagonists have more convincing outcome data when used as initial therapy. It is important to remember that the majority of patients require more than one drug to control their blood pressure. The British Hypertension Society has developed an algorithm for selection of drug therapy – *see* Figure 1.1.

The updated NICE (National Institute for Clinical Excellence) guideline is shown below – *see* Figure 1.2.

Patient profiling

Patients with lipid abnormalities

Small changes in plasma concentrations of cholesterol, triglycerides and LDL cholesterol have been described with large doses of thiazide diuretics. Lower doses produce small and inconsistent changes. Given the clear advantages in terms of cardiovascular outcomes, the recommendation would be to treat lipid abnormalities separately and not to avoid diuretics on the basis of their perceived adverse lipid effects. Triglyceride concentrations increase with selective and non-selective beta-blockers, but the effect on LDL and HDL cholesterol is variable and depends on the drug selected. Lipid abnormalities are not a reason for avoiding beta-adrenoceptor antagonists in hypertension.

Patients with established coronary heart disease

Beta-blockers and calcium-channel antagonists produce symptomatic improvement in patients with angina pectoris (*see* Chapter 2) and should be considered as drugs of first choice. Other antihypertensive agents can improve myocardial oxygen utilisation, however, by lowering blood pressure and decreasing left ventricular hypertrophy.

A number of drugs which are indicated following a myocardial infarction (injury to or death of a section of heart muscle following sudden deprivation of blood supply) – beta-blockers, ACE inhibitors, angiotensin-receptor antagonists and aldosterone antagonists – have antihypertensive activity.

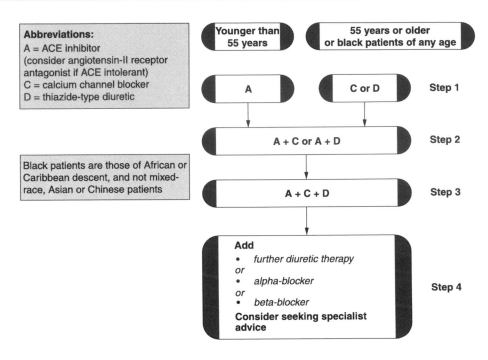

Abbreviations:
A = ACE inhibitor
(consider angiotensin-II receptor
antagonist if ACE intolerant)
C = calcium channel blocker
D = thiazide-type diuretic

Black patients are those of African or
Caribbean descent, and not mixed-
race, Asian or Chinese patients

Younger than 55 years	55 years or older or black patients of any age	
A	C or D	Step 1
A + C or A + D		Step 2
A + C + D		Step 3

Add
- *further diuretic therapy*
or
- *alpha-blocker*
or
- *beta-blocker*

Consider seeking specialist advice

Step 4

Beta-blockers
- Beta-blockers are no longer preferred as a routine initial therapy for hypertension.
- But consider them for younger people, particularly:
  - women of childbearing potential
  - patients with evidence of increased sympathetic drive
  - patients with intolerance of or contraindications to ACE inhibitors and angiotensin-II receptor antagonists.
- If a patient taking a beta-blocker needs a second drug, add a calcium-channel blocker rather than a thiazide type diuretic, to reduce the patient's risk of developing diabetes.
- If a patient's blood pressure is not controlled by a regimen that includes a beta-blocker (that is, it is still above 140/90 mmHg), change their treatment by following the flow chart above.
- If a patient's blood pressure is well controlled (that is, 140/90 mmHg or less) by a regimen that includes a beta-blocker, consider long-term management at their routine review. There is no absolute need to replace the beta-blocker in this case.
- When withdrawing a beta-blocker, step down the dose gradually.
- Beta-blockers should not usually be withdrawn if a patient has a compelling indication for being treated with one, such as symptomatic angina or a previous myocardial infarction.

Figure 1.2: Choosing drugs to lower blood pressure and reduce cardiovascular risk.

Hypertension in the elderly

Older patients benefit greatly from blood pressure reduction, especially in stroke prevention, and there is now limited evidence that the features of dementia may be delayed. Lowering isolated systolic blood pressure has been shown to be beneficial, and interventions which are particularly beneficial in elderly patients include salt reduction, low-dose diuretics, calcium-channel blockers and the angiotensin-receptor antagonist, losartan.

Hypertension in diabetic patients

As previously stated, blood pressure targets are lower in diabetic patients and there has been a preference for drugs which antagonise the renin–angiotensin system, because of their more favourable metabolic profiles and greater evidence that they reduce proteinuria and the progression of renal failure in diabetic nephropathy. However, patients with diabetes and hypertension often require multiple drug therapy, and blood pressure reduction is more important than the choice of the individual agent. Combinations will often include diuretics, calcium-channel antagonists and beta-blockers.

Commonly used antihypertensive agents

Diuretics

Low-dose thiazide diuretics are widely recommended as first-line agents because of their impressive cardiovascular outcome data and low cost. They combine effectively with most other antihypertensive drugs, especially ACE inhibitors and angiotensin-II-receptor antagonists, although the combination with beta-blockers increases the risk of developing diabetes. Diuretics are particularly valuable in older patients, in Afro-Caribbean patients and in those with isolated systolic hypertension or heart failure. For the majority of patients, thiazide diuretics are preferred to loop diuretics, except in patients receiving large doses of vasodilator drugs, for whom long-acting or multiple short-acting loop diuretics are preferred. Spironolactone is often effective in resistant hypertension, particularly when associated with low renin activity.

Adverse effects and interactions

Thiazide diuretics

Chronic therapy frequently results in hypokalaemia (low plasma potassium concentration), since an increased sodium load presented to the renal collecting tubules results in potassium wasting. Hyponatraemia (low plasma sodium concentration), which is often due to a combination of sodium loss and increased plasma volume, is also common. Hyperglycaemia (raised plasma glucose concentration), hyperuricaemia (raised plasma uric acid concentration) with gout and minor lipid abnormalities also occur.

Loop diuretics

Prolonged use of loop diuretics can induce a hypokalaemic metabolic alkalosis. Large doses, when used to treat oedematous conditions (tissue swelling due to fluid retention), can cause hypovolaemia (low blood volume) and hypotension. Ototoxicity and nephrotoxity are more likely to occur in patients with severe renal impairment.

Potassium-sparing diuretics

Hyperkalaemia is the most important adverse effect. Care needs to be exercised when these drugs are combined with other agents that cause potassium retention, e.g. ACE inhibitors, angiotensin-II-receptor antagonists. Spironolactone can cause endocrine abnormalities, e.g. gynaecomastia, testicular atrophy in males and hirsutism in females.

Table 1.1: Interactions with loop and thiazide diuretics

Lithium	Reduced renal clearance of lithium and increased risk of lithium toxicity
Non-steroidal anti-inflammatory drugs	Reduced diuretic and antihypertensive effects
ACE inhibitors	Prior use of diuretics predisposes to first-dose hypotension
Digoxin	Diuretic-induced hypokalaemia increases the risk of digoxin toxicity
Uricosuric agents and xanthine oxidase inhibitors	Reduce the effectiveness of anti-gout medication
Aminoglycosides	Increase the risk of nephrotoxicity when administered together*

*Loop diuretics only.
Source: Johnston GD. *Fundamentals of Cardiovascular Pharmacology.* Chichester: John Wiley & Sons; 1999. p. 136.

For brief descriptions of drug groups, *see British National Formulary (BNF).* For mechanisms of drug action, *see How Drugs Work* (2e) using the Index to locate individual names.

Beta-adrenoceptor antagonists

For more than three decades, beta-blockers have been the drugs of first choice in the treatment of hypertension. Their position as first-line agents has recently been challenged following a number of comparative outcome trials in which beta-blockers (mostly atenolol) have produced disappointing results. The case against beta-blockers is based on two principal factors – they have been shown to be less effective in elderly patients for reducing cardiovascular outcomes, and they are associated with increased evidence of diabetes, especially when combined with diuretics. The current advice from the British Hypertension Society and the National Institute for Clinical Excellence is that beta-blockers are no longer considered first-line agents for the treatment of uncomplicated hypertension. However, they are the drugs of first choice if the patient has angina pectoris or heart failure, or has sustained a previous myocardial infarction. There is little evidence against beta-blockers in patients under 55 years, and in those with high sympathetic activity they remain a satisfactory choice.

Adverse effects and interactions

Several of the adverse effects of beta-blockers are extensions of their known pharmacological effects – bradycardia (slow heart rate), heart block and heart failure. Patients with airways obstruction may deteriorate with beta-blockade. Non-selective beta-blockers have been reported to blunt the clinical manifestations of hypoglycaemia, and effects on the central nervous system can include sedation, fatigue and sleep disturbance, especially if they are lipid soluble.

The combination of beta-blockers with class I anti-arrhythmic drugs can cause severe cardiac depression. Verapamil, diltiazem and cardiac glycosides further depress atrioventricular conduction and can cause bradycardia and heart block. The risk of developing diabetes is increased if beta-blockers are combined with thiazide diuretics. Sudden increases in heart rate and blood pressure can occur following drug withdrawal, sometimes accompanied by prolonged chest pain. Rebound hypertension is more common if clonidine is co-administered, probably due to up-regulation of the beta-receptors (*see How Drugs Work* (2e), Chapter 6).

Calcium-channel blockers

Calcium-channel blockers are now the drugs of first choice in the treatment of hypertension (see ACD rule). They are particularly effective in reducing stroke in older patients with systolic hypertension. ACE inhibitors and diuretics are preferred to calcium-channel antagonists in patients with or at risk of developing heart failure.

Adverse effects and interactions

Calcium-channel blockers, particularly dihydropyridines like amlodipine and nicardipine, cause peripheral oedema, flushing and palpitations. Rate-limiting calcium-channel blockers, such as verapamil and diltiazem, are more likely to cause constipation, heart failure and depression of nodal tissue within the heart. Interactions with beta-blockers, digoxin and anti-arrhythmic agents can result in heart failure and heart block.

Angiotensin-converting-enzyme inhibitors

Angiotensin-converting-enzyme inhibitors are included in the ACD algorithm proposed by the British Hypertension Society for patients under 55 years of age. They combine effectively with diuretics and calcium-channel blockers, and have additional advantages in patients with poor left ventricular function and in those at high cardiovascular risk. They are the drugs of first choice in diabetic hypertensive patients with nephropathy. However, they should be avoided in women of childbearing age, because of potential teratogenicity (foetal abnormalities).

Adverse effects and interactions

The three most important adverse effects of angiotensin-converting-enzyme inhibitors are cough, first-dose hypotension and acute renal impairment. Captopril at high dose was associated with neutropenia, proteinuria and severe allergic reactions when first introduced, but these are rarely reported with currently recommended doses. Cough is the most common adverse effect, occurring in at least 5% of treated patients. It is persistent, non-productive, and more common in women and non-smokers. Hypertensive patients who develop first-dose hypotension and renal impairment have underlying venovascular disease or are volume depleted as a result of previous intensive diuretic therapy. For these reasons, adverse effects are most commonly seen in patients with heart failure and generalised athero-sclerosis. ACE inhibitors decrease the release of aldosterone from the adrenal cortex, and serum potassium levels tend to rise. This is particularly important if renal function is impaired or when other drugs, e.g. potassium-sparing diuretics, angiotensin-II-receptor antagonists, potassium supplements, are given concurrently. Non-steroidal anti-inflammatory drugs blunt the anti-hypertensive effect of ACE inhibitors and other antihypertensive agents, and the combination is particularly problematical in patients with chronic renal impairment. Acute renal failure is likely to occur due to blockade of two important auto-regulatory mechanisms – the renin–angiotensin and renal prostaglandin systems.

Angiotensin-II-receptor antagonists

Angiotensin-II-receptor antagonists should be considered for patients who require an ACE inhibitor but have developed a persistent cough. The evidence for angiotensin-II-receptor antagonists in type 2 diabetes with nephropathy is superior to that for ACE inhibitors.

Adverse effects and interactions

Angiotensin-II-receptor antagonists are a very well tolerated group of compounds with an overall incidence of adverse effects and withdrawals due to adverse effects similar to those for placebo. Cough is no more common than for placebo, and first-dose hypotension and acute renal impairment appear to be less common than with earlier ACE inhibitors. This group of agents is also contraindicated in pregnancy, and the only important interactions occur with drugs that increase the serum potassium level.

Alpha-adrenoceptor antagonists

Since the publication of the ALLHAT study, in which the alpha-blocker was found to be less effective than the diuretic in reducing stroke and heart failure, alpha-blockers are now third- or fourth-line agents in the treatment of hypertension. Since they improve urinary flow in patients with prostatic hypertrophy, they could be used as first-line agents in hypertensive patients with this condition.

Adverse effects and interactions

Most adverse effects of alpha-adrenoceptor antagonists are extensions of their pharmacological properties – hypotension, headache, nasal congestion and impaired ejaculation. First-dose hypotension is more common with prazosin than with longer-acting preparations such as doxazosin and terazosin. Urinary incontinence, particularly in women with uterine prolapse, can be made worse by this group of compounds. Excessive blood pressure reduction with diuretics, calcium-channel blockers and organic nitrates is the most common interaction.

2 Angina pectoris

Pathophysiology

Angina pectoris is a distressing symptom resulting from temporary shortage of blood flow to the heart muscle (myocardial ischaemia). Patients may describe it as pain, tightness, pressure, aching or choking, mainly in the middle front of the chest. Angina is usually brought on by exertion and relieved by resting, but in severe cases, may occur at rest. The discomfort may 'radiate' into the left or right shoulder, arm, wrist, jaw or neck.

The heart requires a large and continuous supply of oxygen to maintain normal cardiac function. To achieve this, a very plentiful blood supply is required. Since oxygen extraction from blood passing through the left ventricle is almost maximal, increased myocardial oxygen demand has to be met by increases in coronary blood flow. On the other hand, decreases in blood flow or increased oxygen demand without increases in oxygen supply will result in myocardial ischaemia. The two determinants of coronary blood flow are the perfusion pressure or inflow pressure for coronary flow and the coronary vascular resistance. Inflow pressure varies markedly throughout the cardiac cycle, due to changes in aortic pressure and the variation in myocardial contractility. Three principal factors influence coronary vascular resistance, namely blood viscosity, the length of the vessel and the diameter of the lumen. Advanced atherosclerosis interferes with the regulation of coronary blood flow by adding fixed resistance in series with the resistance vessels and vasoconstriction beyond the area of stenosis.

In most clinical situations, drug therapy has little or no effect on coronary blood flow. Vasodilator drugs may sometimes improve regional flow to ischaemic areas, and probably account for most of the beneficial effects in

15

patients with chest pain due to coronary artery spasm. The main effect of beta-adrenoceptor antagonists is to reduce oxygen consumption due to reduced heart rate, improved diastolic filling and decreases in afterload. Rate-limiting calcium-channel blockers have similar effects, although these drugs may also have an effect in relieving coronary artery spasm. Occasionally, however, angina may increase due to dilating coronary vessels supplying relatively well-perfused myocardium thus reducing the perfusion of the narrowed vessels.

Myocardial oxygen requirements increase when there is an increase in heart rate, myocardial contractility, arterial blood pressure or ventricular volume (*see* Figure 2.1). Basal metabolic rate, activation of contraction and fibre shortening and the thickness of the ventricular wall also play a part. Most anti-anginal drugs work by reducing myocardial oxygen demand, but in some situations vasodilator drugs can increase oxygen supply.

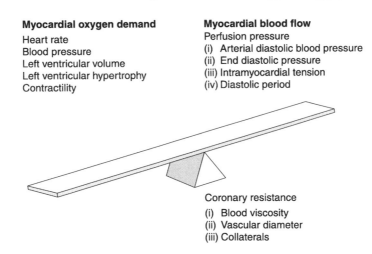

Myocardial oxygen demand
Heart rate
Blood pressure
Left ventricular volume
Left ventricular hypertrophy
Contractility

Myocardial blood flow
Perfusion pressure
(i)   Arterial diastolic blood pressure
(ii) End diastolic pressure
(iii) Intramyocardial tension
(iv) Diastolic period

Coronary resistance
(i)   Blood viscosity
(ii) Vascular diameter
(iii) Collaterals

Figure 2.1: Factors influencing myocardial supply and demand.

Organic nitrates

Glyceryl trinitrate and other short-acting nitrates have been the mainstay of treatment of angina pectoris for over a century. The therapeutic effects of relieving chest pain last for about 30 minutes, so there have been various formulations produced to prolong the anti-anginal effects of organic nitrates. Oral, chewable, transdermal, transmucosal and intravenous forms are now available.

All patients with angina pectoris should receive sublingual or buccal aerosol glyceryl trinitrate for treatment and diagnosis. Rapid relief of chest pain with these preparations strongly supports the diagnosis of angina pectoris. The drug should be taken as early as possible after the onset of angina, or preferably used prophylactically before engaging in activities which are likely to cause chest pain.

Despite extensive first-pass hepatic metabolism, isosorbide dinitrate administered orally improves exercise tolerance for up to 3 hours following a single dose, and for 5 hours during chronic therapy. Isosorbide mononitrate is not subject to significant first-pass metabolism in the liver, so the plasma concentrations are less variable and the optimum therapeutic range is narrower. A large number of oral preparations with these two ingredients, including slow-release compounds, are available for long-term prophylaxis. Intravenous glyceryl trinitrate and isosorbide dinitrate are reserved for the treatment of severe unstable angina, but there are no therapeutic indications for using transdermal preparations. Nitrate tolerance is most likely to occur with these two formulations (see below).

Adverse effects and interactions

Most of the adverse effects of organic nitrates – orthostatic hypotension, tachycardia and headache – are due to excessive vasodilatation. The most important interactions are with other vasodilator drugs, including alcohol and sildenafil (Viagra) and other erection enhancers.

Nitrate tolerance

Nitrate tolerance occurs when continuous administration results in reduced effectiveness. It has been demonstrated in angina pectoris, heart failure and in the peripheral vasculature. It occurs most commonly following continuous intravenous infusion and when long-acting transdermal patches are used, but has also been reported with oral therapy. Studies in patients with angina and heart failure suggest that if plasma nitrate levels are sub-therapeutic for a period of 8 hours, tolerance does not appear to develop. This has led to the introduction of nitrate dosage regimens which include a 'nitrate-free interval', but this is not without its problems. Increased angina has been reported during this time, and it is important to maximise other anti-anginal therapy to ensure good control during this time.

Explanations of nitrate tolerance include receptor down-regulation due to sulfhydryl group depletion (a chemical group of sulfur and hydrogen), neurohormonal activation, plasma volume expansion and increased free radical activity. Interventions other than the 'nitrate-free interval' to reduce nitrate tolerance have been largely unsuccessful.

Nitrate tolerance has been shown to be less with nicorandil, a drug which combines two vasodilator mechanisms – potassium-channel activation and increased cyclic GMP production in vascular smooth muscle.

Beta-adrenoceptor antagonists

Beta-adrenoceptor antagonists are used in the treatment of angina pectoris because they reduce myocardial oxygen demand by decreasing heart rate, myocardial contractility and systemic blood pressure, especially after exercise. Although they remain first-line treatment for the long-term symptomatic management of angina pectoris, almost one in five patients fail to respond.

Choice of beta-blocker

All drugs which block the $beta_1$-receptors are equally effective in the treatment of angina pectoris, provided that equipotent doses are chosen. However, two properties may affect the choice of therapy – $beta_1$ selectivity and partial agonist activity. Overall, $beta_1$-selective drugs are better tolerated, but no clear symptomatic benefit has been described when compared with non-selective agents. Since drugs with partial agonist activity, e.g. pindolol, can increase resting heart rate, they should be avoided in patients with angina at rest.

Adverse effects and interactions

Beta-blockers are more likely to precipitate heart failure and heart block in patients with angina pectoris compared with those with uncomplicated hypertension. Similarly, combinations of beta-blockers with other anti-arrhythmic drugs, especially class I agents and rate-limiting calcium-channel blockers, are more likely to cause heart failure and slow heart rhythms in patients with symptomatic coronary heart disease.

Calcium-channel blockers

All currently available calcium-channel blockers are effective in the long-term management of chronic stable angina. However, when used as monotherapy the rate-limiting drugs diltiazem and verapamil are more effective than the dihydropyridines, such as nifedipine and amlodipine. In addition, aggravation of chest pain is more likely to occur with nifedipine, probably due to reflex increases in heart rate. In contrast, a combination of a beta-blocker with a dihydropyridine calcium-channel blocker is effective in the management of angina pectoris, and is less likely to cause conduction problems than a combination of a beta-blocker and a rate-limiting agent.

Adverse effects and interactions

Apart from worsening angina in a small number of individuals, dihydropyridines are less likely to cause serious cardiac problems than rate-limiting drugs such as verapamil and diltiazem in patients with angina pectoris. Verapamil is the drug most likely to precipitate heart failure, and verapamil and diltiazem can cause serious conduction problems in the Wolff–Parkinson–White syndrome and in patients with first-degree heart block. This is most likely to occur when they are combined with other drugs that reduce heart rate and delay conduction, such as beta-blockers and the I_f-channel inhibitor ivabradine.

I_f-channel inhibitors

A new group of drugs have recently been introduced which act directly on the sinoatrial node (the cardiac pacemaker). At present ivabradine is licensed for the treatment of angina pectoris in patients with normal sinus rhythm (> 60 beats/minute) when beta-blockers are contraindicated or poorly tolerated.

Adverse effects and contraindications

The principal adverse effects are cardiac arrhythmias, bradycardia and first-degree heart block. Visual disturbances, vertigo and muscle cramps will limit the use of this group of compounds. Problems are likely to be made worse if ivabradine is combined with other drugs that cause bradycardia and delay cardiac conduction, namely beta-blockers and rate-limiting calcium-channel blockers.

3 Acute coronary syndrome

The term 'acute coronary syndrome' is now used to describe a number of conditions which present with chest pain due to acute myocardial ischaemia. When the condition results in myocardial injury it is termed myocardial infarction. The acute coronary syndrome also includes ST-elevation myocardial infarction (STEMI), non-ST-elevation myocardial infarction (NSTEMI) and unstable angina. ST elevation refers to the elevation above the baseline of the final two sections of the electrocardiograph (ECG) trace of the cardiac contraction wave, PQRST.

- STEMI is an acute coronary syndrome where patients present with ischaemic chest pain and ST-segment elevation on the ECG, and for which reperfusion treatment is essential.
- NSTEMI is an acute coronary syndrome that is not associated with ST-segment elevation but with evidence of myocardial injury as assessed by elevated cardiac muscle enzymes.
- Unstable angina is an acute coronary syndrome without ST-segment changes and without evidence of myocardial injury.

Only patients with STEMI should receive thrombolysis.

Drug treatment of ST-elevation myocardial infarction

Initial management

All patients should have ECG monitoring in an environment where defibrillation and pacing can be performed. Aspirin 300 mg should be given to all patients unless there are clear contraindications. Intramuscular injections should be avoided because of the increased muscle enzyme activity and high risk of bleeding if thrombolytics are administered.

Control of pain

Diamorphine administered intravenously is generally considered to be the drug of first choice unless severe hypotension and/or respiratory depression are present. Metoclopramide is probably the safest anti-emetic for reducing opiate-induced nausea and vomiting.

Oxygen

Ventilation/perfusion abnormalities occur secondary to pulmonary oedema and associated hypoxaemia, and require treatment with oxygen.

Nitrates

Sublingual or intravenous organic nitrates can be used to reduce chest pain provided that the patient is not hypotensive. Particular caution is required in right ventricular infarcts, as venodilatation can precipitate severe hypotension. Nitrates have no effect on mortality.

Beta-adrenoceptor antagonists

Early administration of a beta-blocker reduces infarct size and life-threatening arrhythmias. Patients with elevated blood pressure, tachycardia, atrial fibrillation and recurrent chest pain are most likely to benefit, while those with bradycardia, hypotension and conduction problems are most likely to experience adverse effects.

ACE inhibitors

ACE inhibitors or the angiotensin-II-receptor antagonist valsartan should also be administered within 24 hours after an ST-elevation infarction or for those with left bundle branch block. Most benefit is due to improvement in left ventricular function.

Thrombolytic agents: clot-busters

For patients with ST-segment elevation, thrombolysis results in reperfusion in 50–70% of those treated. This is translated into improved left ventricular function, and reduced arrhythmias, cardiogenic shock and mortality. The best results occur if percutaneous coronary intervention is performed soon after drug administration. The greatest benefit is achieved with early thrombolysis, especially if given within 4 hours of the onset of chest pain.

Streptokinase

Streptokinase is the most commonly used thrombolytic agent in the UK. Antistreptococcal antibodies are commonly present, and the dose must be sufficient to overcome their effects.

Adverse effects and contraindications

Bleeding, symptomatic hypotension and allergic reactions are the most common and serious reactions associated with streptokinase therapy. However, hypertension can be associated with reperfusion, due to successful thrombolysis and recanalisation. Allergic reactions – which include fever, rashes, serum sickness, polyneuropathy and (rarely) anaphylaxis (an allergic

Table 3.1: Advantages and disadvantages of the three commonly available thrombolytic agents

Drug	Advantages	Disadvantages
Streptokinase	Clinically proven value Relatively inexpensive	Antigenic Occasional allergic reaction Hypotension
Anistreplase	Clinically proven value Rapid effect with prolonged action	Antigenic Occasional allergic reaction Moderately expensive
Alteplase	Clinically proven value Non-antigenic Highly clot selective	Simultaneous heparin therapy required Short half-life Very expensive

emergency) – occur in about 12% of patients treated. These reactions are rarely seen with other thrombolytic agents, e.g. alteplase, and severe reactions usually occur on re-exposure. Any condition which increases the risk of bleeding represents a relative or absolute contraindication to the use of streptokinase and other thrombolytic agents. A previous history of an allergic reaction to streptokinase is an absolute contraindication. Great care is also required when giving thrombolytic drugs to patients who are already receiving anticoagulants and antiplatelet drugs.

Clopidogrel

All patients following an acute coronary syndrome or who have undergone percutaneous coronary intervention should receive clopidogrel. A loading dose of 300 mg followed by a maintenance dose of 75 mg was the regimen used in the outcome trials. This should be combined with 75 mg of aspirin to reduce platelet aggregation and thereby the clotting mechanism. To date there is no evidence of clinical benefit beyond 1 year for the combination.

Treatment of non-ST-elevation myocardial infarction and unstable angina

The treatment of NSTEMI/unstable angina differs from that of STEMI in a number of key areas:

- Thrombolytic therapy is of no proven value.
- Rate-limiting calcium-channel blockers such as verapamil or diltiazem are useful adjuvants to analgesics, nitrates and beta-blockers.
- HMG CoA reductase inhibitors (the statins) have been shown to reduce mortality and recurrent myocardial infarction when administered in the acute setting.
- Glycoprotein-IIb/IIIa (e.g. eptifibatide and tirofiban, for specialist use only) antagonists have been shown to protect patients with NSTEMI and unstable angina from death and non-fatal myocardial infarction during the acute phase of their presentation and for 24 hours following intervention.
- Unfractionated and low-molecular-weight heparin reduces the risk of further myocardial infarction, often combined with antiplatelet drugs.

4 Heart failure

Heart failure covers a spectrum of conditions ranging from asymptomatic reduced left ventricular function to symptomatic ventricular failure at rest. In pathophysiological terms it can be defined as the inability of the heart to deliver blood and hence oxygen at a rate necessary for adequate tissue metabolism, despite normal or elevated ventricular filling pressures. This definition implies a primary defect in systolic function, although diastolic dysfunction is present in almost half of the patients with heart failure. In addition, salt and water retention, peripheral vasoconstriction and increased heart rate occur secondary to neurohormonal activation, which can further impair tissue oxygenation. Clinical heart failure is defined as a syndrome characterised by dyspnoea, fatigue and oedema occurring as a consequence of inadequate oxygen delivery and elevated filling pressure. In a small number of patients with reduced left ventricular function, these features may be absent and fatigue is the predominant feature.

Pathophysiology

The changes which occur in heart failure can be considered in terms of three major determinants – contractility, pre-load and after-load.

Contractility

This is defined as the force with which the left ventricle can contract independent of heart rate, pre-load and after-load. Impaired contractility is due not only to loss of functioning muscle but also to abnormal responses in surviving muscle, probably induced by neurohormonal activation.

Pre-load

This describes the relationship between end-diastolic fibre stretch and muscle function. These are assessed indirectly by measuring the left ventricular end-diastolic pressure and the stroke volume (or cardiac output). The relationship between these two measurements is known as the Frank–Starling curve (*see* Figure 4.1). In heart failure the left ventricular function curve is much flatter, and an increase in pre-load produces little change in cardiac output. As the end-diastolic pressure increases, the risk of pulmonary oedema also increases (*see* Figure 4.1).

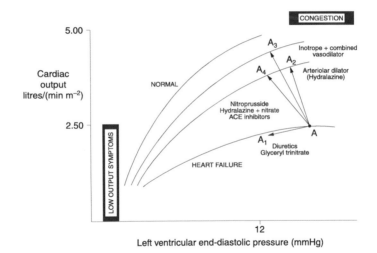

Figure 4.1: The effects of cardiovascular drugs on the Frank–Starling relationship in heart failure.

After-load

This refers to the tension or force per unit cross-sectional area in the wall of the ventricle during ejection of blood from the ventricle. It is mostly determined by systemic vascular resistance, but large artery compliance, blood viscosity and intra-arterial blood volume also play a part. The failing heart is very sensitive to increases in after-load, so peripheral vasoconstriction induced by activation of the sympathetic and renin–angiotensin system can result in marked decreases in cardiac output. Conversely, a small decrease in after-load, produced by vasodilator drugs, can substantially increase cardiac output.

Rationale for the use of drugs in congestive cardiac failure

There are three main areas of therapeutic intervention in the treatment of heart failure:

1 diuretics to reduce plasma volume and venous pressure
2 vasodilators to increase venous capacitance and reduce after-load
3 drugs to modulate inotropic (the force with which the heart contracts) function.

Short-term benefit can be achieved with positive inotropic agents, but long-term use is associated with increased mortality. Beta-adrenoceptor agents which reduce heart rate, blood pressure and inotropic function have been shown to increase life expectancy and reduce hospital admissions.

The use of diuretics in heart failure

Most patients with heart failure have elevated left ventricular end-diastolic volume for a given ventricular performance. The inability of cardiac output to increase with effort results in under-perfusion of the tissues with increased fatigue and exertional dyspnoea. The kidney responds by increasing sodium and water uptake by the renal tubule, and the plasma volume increases. Ultimately pulmonary vascular congestion results and movement of fluid from the pulmonary capillaries into the alveoli causes pulmonary oedema.

Diuretics produce their beneficial effects by reducing plasma volume and venous return to the heart. Loop diuretics are the preferred agents since they have steep dose–response relationships, produce acute venodilation and increase renal blood flow independent of their diuretic effects. A fall in blood pressure due to decreased after-load can also improve cardiac haemodynamics.

The use of vasodilator drugs in heart failure

The rationale for using vasodilator drugs in the treatment of heart failure came initially from observations with sodium nitroprusside in acute heart failure, when cardiac output increased markedly with reductions in pre-load and after-load. However, long-term studies with conventional vasodilators produced variable results. Most produced symptomatic improvement and better quality of life. A combination of hydralazine and isosorbide dinitrate reduced mortality in heart failure, the alpha-blocker prazosin and direct-acting vasodilators had no effect, while most calcium-channel antagonists were less effective than placebo.

Since 1987, following the publication of the CONSENSUS study, angiotensin-converting-enzyme (ACE) inhibitors have remained the vasodilator drugs of first choice in the management of heart failure. They have been shown to produce symptomatic improvement and to prolong life expectancy in all grades of heart failure, and to delay the development of symptomatic heart failure in patients with reduced left ventricular systolic function. ACE inhibitors have a number of actions which could impact on this favourable response. They do reduce pre-load and after-load without increasing heart rate. They reverse the detrimental haemodynamic effects induced by increased circulating and tissue levels of angiotensin II and aldosterone. Finally, their effects on cardiac volume, structure, pressures, electrolyte balance and autonomic function are likely to have an important impact on the development of arrhythmias.

The use of inotropes in the treatment of heart failure

The main aim of inotropic therapy is to provide support for the heart to maintain adequate oxygen perfusion. This can be achieved in low-output or congestive cardiac failure for short periods, but long-term beneficial effects are more difficult to demonstrate and mortality tends to increase. Tolerance, increased risks of arrhythmias and down-regulation of the beta-receptors have all been suggested as explanations. Digitalis remains the only inotropic drug which is recommended for general clinical use. A recent large outcome trial demonstrated that digoxin had no beneficial or detrimental effects on mortality, but did reduce hospital admissions due to worsening heart failure.

Digoxin

Clinical use

Digitalis remains the treatment of choice when heart failure is accompanied by fast atrial fibrillation. Conversion from atrial fibrillation to sinus rhythm rarely occurs. In patients with heart failure and sinus rhythm, the main beneficial effects are seen in those with markedly impaired systolic function and those who are already receiving diuretics, ACE inhibitors and spirono-lactone. Within the therapeutic range there is no clear evidence of a dose–response relationship.

Adverse effects and interactions

The adverse effects of digoxin are well documented and can be divided into three groups, namely gastrointestinal effects, cardiac dysrhythmias and neurological effects. Important gastrointestinal effects include anorexia, nausea and vomiting, and diarrhoea. The most common dysrhythmias are ventricular ectopics (unregulated extra ventricular beats), atrial tachycardia with heart block and various degrees of heart block. Neurological effects, apart from visual disturbances, often go undetected and can include fatigue, general malaise, confusion and disorientation, especially in the elderly.

Table 4.1: Some important cardiovascular drugs which increase the serum digoxin concentration

Drug	Average increase in steady-state plasma concentration (%)
Amiodarone	70–100
Propafenone	25–35
Quinidine	100
Spironolactone	20
Verapamil	50–100

Table 4.2: Factors that increase sensitivity to digoxin and other cardiac glycosides

Underlying pathology
  Cor pulmonale
  Myxoedema
  Chronic rheumatic or viral carditis
  Acute myocardial infarction

Electrolyte disorders
  Hypokalaemia
  Hypomagnesaemia
  Hypercalcaemia

Problems caused by diuretics in heart failure

Reduction of the extracellular fluid volume is a common complication of loop diuretics in heart failure. Volume depletion can lead to impaired renal function and contribute to the metabolic alkalosis which often accompanies diuretic-induced hypokalaemia. In the past, the commonest complication of loop diuretics was hypokalaemia, which increased the risk of digitalis-induced arrhythmias, but with the introduction of ACE inhibitors, angiotensin-receptor antagonists and spironolactone to the treatment of heart failure, hyperkalaemia is now a more common problem. Hyponatraemia is now the commonest electrolyte abnormality that occurs in heart failure, and further reductions can occur with a high fluid intake. This is in part related to increased anti-diuretic hormone (ADH) release secondary to volume contraction. Acute urinary retention in men with prostatic hypertrophy is relatively common, particularly after intravenous administration.

Problems caused by ACE inhibitors in heart failure

Symptomatic hypotension following ACE inhibition is a common problem in heart failure. It is most likely to occur in severe heart failure when the initial blood pressure is low and the patient is volume-contracted as a result of intensive diuretic therapy. Acute deterioration in renal function also occurs more commonly in these patients, especially if renovascular disease is present.

Problems caused by inotropes in heart failure

Inotropes can be used to provide short-term support in patients with low-output cardiac failure, but long-term beneficial effects are more difficult to demonstrate and mortality increases. Since advanced heart failure is a state of energy starvation in which catecholamine activity (particularly adrenaline and noradrenaline) is high and the beta-receptors are down-regulated, it seems likely that further stimulation would be unsuccessful or even harmful. Digitalis remains the only inotrope which is recommended for general clinical use, although no beneficial effects on mortality have been described.

The role of beta-adrenoceptor antagonists

A number of clinical outcome trials have confirmed the benefit of a number of beta-adrenoceptor antagonists, namely metoprolol, bisoprolol, carvedilol and nebivolol. The main benefit is due to a reduction in mortality and hospitalisations due to heart failure. It is important to start with a very small dose and titrate upwards slowly, since the drop-out rate due to fatigue and worsening heart failure will be high if large doses are introduced at the beginning of treatment. Start low and go slow.

Conclusion

It will have been obvious that few medical conditions require greater caution in selecting an optimal drug regimen for the individual patient than heart failure. The likelihood of benefit must be balanced against the strong possibility of harm. Such patients require regular on-going shared care with a consultant cardiologist.

5 Hyperlipidaemia and cardiovascular risk

Dyslipidaemia (abnormal blood fats) refers to all abnormalities of lipid metabolism (manufacture and removal of blood fats). Hyperlipoproteinaemia includes those conditions in which lipoprotein levels are increased, e.g. increased low-density lipoproteins (LDL). Hypercholesterolaemia is a condition in which total and LDL-cholesterol levels are increased but the levels of triglycerides (natural fats) are normal. Mixed hyperlipidaemia refers to high LDL-cholesterol levels with low high-density lipoprotein (HDL) cholesterol and increased triglycerides. The terms 'high-density' and 'low-density' lipoprotein refer to layers formed in a test tube when plasma samples are spun at very high speed in a centrifuge (ultracentrifugation).

Management of lipid abnormalities and prevention of cardiovascular disease

Accelerated development of atherosclerosis (hardening of the arteries) is strongly associated with increased concentrations of LDL cholesterol and reduced concentrations of HDL cholesterol. Increased triglycerides probably also contribute, but the effect is small and related to associated low HDL-cholesterol levels. The impact of these lipid abnormalities is influenced by other cardiovascular risk factors, such as age, cigarette smoking, diabetes, hypertension and a positive family history of coronary heart disease and stroke. All patients with established heart disease, stroke or peripheral vascular disease should receive a statin – simvastatin, pravastatin or atorvastatin (secondary prevention) – and patients with risk factors for cardiovascular disease but without established disease should have their cardiovascular risk assessed using the charts at the back of the *British National Formulary*. These charts estimate the 10-year risk of developing coronary heart disease or stroke based on age, gender, systolic blood pressure, and the ratio of total cholesterol to HDL cholesterol. Smoking, family history of stroke or heart disease, elevated triglyceride levels, premature menopause, impaired glucose tolerance and certain ethnic groups all increase the risk further, and these should be included in the assessment. Patients who have a 20% risk or higher should normally receive a statin (primary prevention). Risk tables are not suitable for patients with diabetes, and those with diabetes who are over 40 years of age should receive a statin.

Lifestyle interventions to reduce cardiovascular disease

Table 5.1: Joint British Societies Guidelines 2005

Lifestyle targets

1 Do not smoke.
2 Maintain ideal body weight for adults (body mass index 20–25 kg/m^2) and avoid central obesity (waist circumference in white Caucasians should be < 102 cm in men and < 88 cm in women, and in Asians < 90 cm in men and < 80 cm in women).
3 Keep total dietary intake of fat to = 30% of total energy intake.
4 Keep intake of saturated fats to = 10% of total fat intake.
5 Keep intake of dietary cholesterol to < 300 mg/day.
6 Replace saturated fats with an increased intake of monounsaturated fats.
7 Increase intake of fresh fruit and vegetables to at least five portions per day.
8 Regular intake of fish and other sources of omega-3 fatty acids (at least two servings of fish per week).
9 Limit alcohol intake to < 21 units/week for men or < 14 units/week for women.
10 Limit intake of salt to < 100 mmol/l day (< 6 g of sodium chloride or < 2.4 g of sodium per day).
11 Take regular aerobic physical activity for at least 30 minutes per day, most days of the week (e.g. fast walking, swimming).

Selection of drug therapies

Currently available lipid-lowering drugs include statins, fibrates, fish oils and drugs to reduce cholesterol absorption. The statins have the best evidence for preventing heart disease and stroke. They are the most effective for lowering LDL cholesterol, but can increase HDL cholesterol (especially rosuvastatin) and lower triglycerides. They are first-line drugs for lowering LDL cholesterol. Other agents will be needed in some patients when a statin alone is insufficient for reducing LDL cholesterol, when they are intolerant of a statin, or when the triglyceride levels are very high. Fibrates are mainly used for mixed hyperlipidaemia, and can be added to a statin under specialist advice. Ezetimibe reduces cholesterol absorption, is well tolerated and can be added to a statin to achieve the cholesterol target, or used alone in patients who are intolerant of a statin.

Safety of statins

The benefits of statin therapy in large populations greatly outweigh their adverse effects. The two main adverse effects – liver damage and rhabdo-myolysis (breakdown of muscle) – are very rare with currently available statins. These adverse effects are more common when statins are combined with fibrates (especially gemfibrozil). See *BNF* for recommended liver function testing.

Lipid treatment targets

There is at present no general agreement on the targets for primary and secondary prevention. A target of less than 5 mmol/l total cholesterol and/or 3 mmol/l LDL cholesterol (or a reduction of 30% in either) remains the recommendation within the UK. A number of specialist groups would prefer the lower targets suggested by the Joint British Societies' Guidelines for total cholesterol (< 4 mmol/l) and LDL cholesterol (< 2 mmol/l).

Conclusion

We have now definitely reached an era of preventive medicine with drug therapy. Although stopping smoking, switching to healthier diets and taking increased exercise have an impact on the incidence of cardiovascular disease, drugs to lower cholesterol and blood pressure for primary prevention and aspirin and warfarin in addition for secondary prevention have major additional benefits.

6 Diabetes

Introduction

Diabetes is one of the commonest and most serious chronic diseases, threatening both quality of life and premature death if poorly managed. Once diagnosed, treatment is lifelong and requires regular clinical supervision, with readjustment of the treatment regimen to suit the patient's current needs. Ideally, management of diabetes includes not only drug treatment, but also sustained lifestyle modifications, in particular a balanced diet and regular exercise. It needs the patient's understanding and commitment if it is to succeed. Unfortunately, many diabetics (40–50%) comply poorly with all of these.

Treatment of diabetics should always be planned and coordinated by a medical specialist, whether hospital based or a GP with special interest. For that reason, this chapter will give only a basic outline of treatment. No one without special training in diabetic care (at least a 6-month attachment to a specialist unit) should attempt to manage any diabetic alone. Diabetic specialist nurses now have an important role in ongoing care.

What is diabetes?

Diabetes could be thought of as failure of the body's insulin-secreting organ – the beta cells of the pancreas. Insulin is necessary to regulate the plasma glucose concentration, to supply muscles with their energy source for contraction and to regulate fat metabolism. Insulin deprivation in diabetics causes profound abnormalities of carbohydrate, fat and protein metabolism (details of which can be found in any modern medical physiology textbook). Therein lies the threat to health and life. Good management can restore metabolic near-normality and prevent or reduce the disastrous complications of diabetes, including accelerated damage to large and small arteries, known respectively as macrovascular and microvascular lesions. This has devastating effects on many organs.

1 **Macrovascular disease** (accelerated atheroma) affects:

- the coronary arteries, with a greatly increased risk of early coronary heart disease (CHD), angina pectoris and heart attack (myocardial infarction)
- the cerebral arteries, with an increased risk of stroke (cerebral thrombosis/infarction)
- all of the other large arteries, with an increased risk of blockage by thrombosis, that adds to the problem of:

2 **Microvascular disease**, which affects the small peripheral arteries, leading to.

- hypertension (high blood pressure)
- retinal damage (diabetic retinopathies), leading to blindness if left untreated
- inadequate circulation to the skin, nerves and other tissues of the lower limbs (peripheral ischaemia), leading to gangrene and amputation
- some diabetic neuropathies are due to nerve ischaemia caused by small artery blockage; other diabetic neuropathy is due to lesions of the sensory and motor nerve axons.

Perhaps the most important complication of diabetes is progressive kidney damage – diabetic nephropathy, with loss of many renal glomeruli, micro-albuminuria (leakage of plasma protein into the urine) and, eventually, end-stage renal failure.

All of these complications of diabetes develop slowly over years, so that patients have no warning symptoms of the risks they are incurring by poor compliance until it is too late.

The two types of diabetes – type 1 and type 2

('Type 1' and 'type 2' are the correct modern terms.)

Type 1 diabetes may be considered as 'acute beta-cell failure', in which an unknown disease process destroys all beta cells in the pancreas, leading to an absolute insulin deficit. It is commonest in children and adolescents, particularly those with a first-degree (immediate family) type 1 diabetic relative. When 90% of the beta cells have been destroyed, the patient presents with:

- polydipsia (excessive thirst and fluid consumption)
- polyuria (excessive excretion of dilute urine)
- weight loss despite normal appetite
- often a faint smell of acetone on the patient's breath.

   On testing the urine and blood, there is usually:

- glucose in the urine (glycosuria)
- ketone in the urine (ketonuria)
- fasting blood glucose concentration in excess of 7 mmol/1 on consecutive days (hyperglycaemia)
- impaired oral glucose tolerance test – plasma glucose concentration in excess of 11 mmol/1, 2 hours after drinking a solution containing 75 grams of glucose on a fasting stomach.

   The first presentation of type 1 diabetes is often a medical emergency which needs immediate hospitalization in a specialist unit, with insulin treatment followed by stabilization on insulin, advice on diet and lifestyle by the diabetic team, and education of the patient (and parents, if appropriate) being of great importance. There is a risk of hyperglycaemic coma (due to excessively high plasma glucose levels) and death.

   Type 2 diabetes may be thought of as 'chronic beta-cell failure', with a gradual, progressive reduction in insulin secretion and a resulting rise in plasma glucose levels (hyperglycaemia). This deficit is usually accompanied by tissue insensitivity to insulin action, with cause unknown (insulin resistance). There may be no symptoms, which is why clinicians must actively seek the diagnosis, particularly in obese older patients with a family history of diabetes, and those with raised serum triglyceride levels in a serum lipid estimation. On questioning, the patient may admit to fatigue ('I'm tired all the time'), some loss of visual acuity (easily confirmed by an eye chart) and ano-genital itching (due to thrush infection). Type 2 diabetes is more common in women who have had diabetes during pregnancy, and in people of Asian and Afro-Caribbean origin who have adopted a western diet. The same clinical tests as for type 1 diabetes will confirm the diagnosis, including (essentially) a glucose tolerance test. In addition, the condensation of glucose on the haemoglobin in red blood cells is proportional to the concentration of glucose in the blood, and is monitored as the haemoglobin A_{1c} (HbA$_{1c}$) (check the upper limit of normal with your area laboratory). It is a useful check on an individual patient's longer-term diabetic control.

The concept of pre-diabetes

This is a state of impaired glucose tolerance and raised fasting blood glucose concentration. At a time when clinical practice is shifting towards pro-active/ pre-emptive care, it is important to realize that a reduction in insulin secretion and the development of insulin resistance with increasing hyper-glycaemia probably occur gradually over a decade before type 2 diabetes is diagnosed. This can be revealed by an oral glucose tolerance test in the type of patients just described, when a 2-hour plasma glucose concentration of 8–11 mmol/1 is diagnostic. (A fasting plasma glucose concentration of 6–7 mmol/1 should lead at once to an oral glucose tolerance test.) The importance of diagnosing pre-diabetes is that these patients are already incurring the risks of diabetes (see above), which good management will greatly reduce, extending life and maintaining quality of life.

The treatment/management of type 1 diabetes mellitus

The main treatment of type 1 diabetes is the replacement of insulin, supplemented by a balanced, calorie-controlled diet and regular, rhythmic exercise (walking, jogging, cycling, swimming or aerobics, depending on individual ability and preference). Figure 6.1 shows the pattern of normal insulin secretion over 24 hours. Note the rapid onset of high concentrations of insulin within minutes of starting each meal, and the return to baseline concentrations within 3 hours, coinciding with the digestion and absorption of food and the consequent rise in blood glucose, amino acids and fats. Note also that there is a minimum 'background' basal secretion of insulin between meals and at night. **In type 1 diabetes, insulin secretion is zero, or close to zero.** Modern treatment aims to replicate this normality, in so far as that is possible.

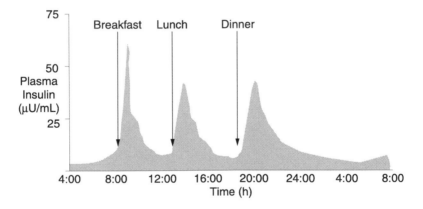

Figure 6.1: Physiological serum insulin secretion profile.

The aim of treatment is to prevent post-prandial (post feeding) hyper-glycaemia and avoid the adverse side-effect of insulin treatment, namely inter-prandial (between meals) hypoglycaemia (particularly nocturnal). This is not always easy in individual patients, as first the dose(s) of insulin have to be determined, and then the optimal combination of injected insulin must be found, which may take weeks or months at the start. All that the beginner needs to know is concisely stated in the *BNF*, Chapter 6.1.1 on 'Insulins', which could hardly be bettered for clarity. Here (reproduced with permission) are two short paragraphs from the *BNF*:

'Insulin preparations can be divided into 3 types:

- those of **short** duration which have a relatively rapid onset of action, namely soluble insulin, insulin lispro and insulin aspart;
- those with an **intermediate** duration of action, e.g. isophane insulin and insulin zinc suspension; and
- those whose action is slower in onset and lasts for **long** periods, e.g. insulin zinc suspension.

The duration of action of a particular type of insulin varies considerably from one patient to another, and needs to be assessed individually.

Examples of recommended insulin regimens:

- Short-acting insulin mixed with intermediate-acting insulin: twice daily (before meals).
- Short-acting insulin mixed with intermediate-acting insulin: before breakfast (and)
  short-acting insulin: before evening meal
  intermediate-acting insulin: at bedtime.
- Short-acting insulin: three times daily (before breakfast, mid-day and evening meal)
  intermediate-acting insulin: at bedtime.
- Intermediate-acting insulin with or without short-acting insulin: once daily either before breakfast or at bedtime suffices for some patients with type 2 diabetes who need insulin.'*

(BNF No. 54, Chapter 6.1.1. September 2007)**

For maintenance therapy, insulins are injected subcutaneously (between the skin and deeper tissues), varying the site of injection from the abdomen to the thighs, upper arms and buttocks. Insulin acts by binding with insulin receptors on the cell surface, activating a cellular enzyme which causes a large increase in glucose transporters (GLUT4) in cell membranes. These carry glucose molecules into the muscle, fat and liver cells (*How Drugs Work*, Chapter 8). Insulin also increases glucose metabolism and synthesis of glycogen (the carbohydrate storage molecule) in muscle. The insulin-

* Sometimes in combination with oral hypoglycaemic drugs (see below).
** For current *BNF* guidelines please visit bnf.org.

sensitive/insulin-dependent cells are those of all muscle and adipose (fat) tissue and liver. A further six GLUT-type carriers transport glucose into the remaining body tissues without the presence of insulin.

The importance of exercise in diabetics

Regular, rhythmic, sub-maximal daily exercise substantially reduces the need for injected insulin. *Independent of insulin*, exercise increases the number of GLUT4 glucose transporters in insulin-sensitive tissues, lowering blood glucose levels (this may cause a risk of hypoglycaemia in type 1 diabetics who are unaccustomed to exercise – all diabetics should carry glucose tablets with them day and night).

Regular exercise also trains the heart, lungs and muscles, lowers blood pressure and has a beneficial effect in depressive illness. Exercise should be a major feature of the management plans of most diabetics, whether type 1 or type 2.

The centrality of diet in diabetes

The ideal diet for individual diabetics should be prescribed by a dietitian. It should be high in soluble fibre, low in saturated fats, contain plenty of poultry, fish and veal, and carbohydrate from wholegrain products (for slow release of glucose), and supply no more than the estimated daily calorie requirement. More than 50% of all diabetics comply very poorly with their diet. Those who do comply include those who become skilled in 'calorie counting' – they self-administer 1 unit of insulin lispro for every 10–15 grams of carbohydrate eaten. They also adjust their insulin dosage according to that day's exercise and increase it during infections.

Treatment of type 2 diabetes

The aim of type 2 diabetes treatment is to 'make the most' of what insulin-secreting capacity remains, by means of oral drugs, exercise and diet, and when those fail (due to progressive beta-cell failure), to switch without delay to injected insulin treatment. As with type 1 diabetes, management must be skilfully tailored to individual needs. A stepwise approach is a useful concept (*see* Figure 6.2).

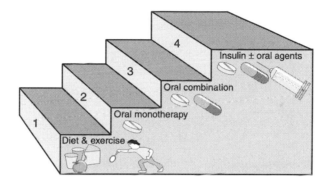

Figure 6.2: Stepwise management of Type 2 diabetes.

Initially, given enthusiastic compliance by the patient, weight loss down to nearly ideal body mass index (BMI), a strict diet (low fat, higher protein and wholegrain carbohydrate, supplying no more than the estimated daily calorie needs) and daily rhythmic exercise (30 minutes of brisk walking or relaxed jogging, swimming or cycling) will reverse the metabolic abnormalities and return the blood glucose profile to almost normal (see above section on metabolic benefits of regular exercise). Some patients achieve this, particularly younger individuals (40–60 years) with pre-diabetes.

More often it is necessary to proceed to Step 2, using a single anti-diabetic (hypoglycaemic) drug, diet and exercise. Because of evidence from the large UKPDS study, metformin is often a good first choice. If that fails, two drugs from different groups (*see* Figure 6.2) are tried, and it may be necessary to try several combinations before the optimal combination is found. If these fail, insulin should be added without delay. Steps 3 and 4 require experience and expertise, and are best learned in the setting of a diabetic clinic.

The oral hypoglycaemic drugs

The creativity and scientific drive of the drug industry have given us a good selection of anti-diabetic drug groups (*see* Table 6.1). Remember that all of

Table 6.1: Oral hypoglycaemic drug groups

Drug group	Examples	Action	Advantages/disadvantages
Biguanide	metformin	Decreases intestinal absorption of glucose Decreases glucose production by liver Increases glucose uptake by skeletal muscle	A good first choice, particularly in obese patients Reduces cardiovascular risk in obese patients *Often causes nausea, anorexia and diarrhoea* *Avoid in CHF, COPD, and renal and hepatic disease**
Sulphonylureas	glibenclamide gliclazide	Close potassium channels on the beta cells, which stimulates insulin secretion (*How Drugs Work*, Chapter 8, Table 8.1)	Well tolerated and effective *Hypoglycaemia is a risk, and can be severe and prolonged with glibenclamide, which should not be used in the elderly* *Stimulate appetite and often cause weight gain* *May interact seriously with alcohol – a disulfiram-like effect (*How Drugs Work*, Chapter 23, paragraph on alcohol)* *Several drugs augment their hypoglycaemic effect increasing the risk of hypoglycaemia (*BNF*, Appendix 1)* Sulphonylureas can be combined with metformin or the glitazones (see below)
Glitazones (thiazolidinediones) NB: see NICE guidance, *BNF*, 6.1.2.3	rosiglitazone pioglitazone	Reduce glucose output by liver Increase glucose uptake by muscle Reduce triglycerides and free fatty acids in plasma	Effective as monotherapy or in combination Not suitable as first-line therapy *Note: Slow onset (1–2 months for maximum effect) Regular liver function tests necessary (possibly hepatotoxic)* *Cause weight gain and fluid retention – do not use in patients with heart or renal failure* *Contraindicated in pregnant and breastfeeding women*

| Alpha-glucosidase | acarbose | Inhibits the action of amylases** and sucrase in the intestine, lowering plasma glucose concentration by reducing its availability | Usually used in combination (effect on blood glucose concentration is small)
Causes marked flatulence (and sometimes colic), as undigested carbohydrate is processed by bacterial flora, producing gases
Causes troublesome diarrhoea in some patients
Some risk of hypoglycaemia in combination with sulphonylureas or insulin |
| Meglitinides | nateglinide repaglinide | Stimulate insulin secretion by pancreatic beta cells – act at same receptor as the sulphonylureas (see above) | Short duration of action, low risk of hypoglycaemia
Can be taken 30 minutes before meals to reduce glucose 'peak' (*see* Figure 6.1) in patients who are well controlled by diet and exercise (monotherapy)
Cause less weight gain than sulphonylureas
Do not use in combination with sulphonylureas
Note: Nateglinide is only licensed for use with metformin
Small risk of hypoglycaemia and hypersensitive rashes/urticaria
Repaglinide may cause abdominal pain, diarrhoea, constipation, nausea and vomiting |

* CHF, congestive heart failure; COPD, chronic obstructive pulmonary disease.

** Enzymes that digest carbohydrates.

these support the patient's remaining insulin output (in different ways), reducing the complications of diabetes and postponing the day when insulin is needed.

The importance of treating hypertension in diabetics

Given adequate diabetic control, the tight regulation of blood pressure greatly reduces a diabetic's risk of accelerated cardiovascular, cerebrovascular, renal and peripheral vascular disease. A target blood pressure of 130/80 mmHg should be the aim, particularly in patients with diabetic kidney disease. However, this usually needs combination therapy of the hypertension (*see* Chapter 1). Add this to the oral hypoglycaemics, insulin, and probably a statin to improve hypercholesterolaemia, and the patient could be required to take six or more tablets per day. It needs an intelligent and highly motivated person to comply adequately with such a regime. Compliance/concordance must be encouraged by all doctors, nurses, pharmacists and dietitians at every opportunity. Remember also the potential of polypharmacy (multiple drug treatment) for serious drug interactions (*see How Drugs Work*, Chapter 23).

Diabetic self-monitoring

Compliance with the treatment regimen is not enough, if a diabetic patient is to maintain optimal control. Regular self-monitoring of plasma glucose levels is essential in type 1 diabetes. This is done using glucose reagent test strips, read by a matching meter. A drop of capillary blood (finger prick) is applied to the strip, which is then placed on or in the meter, which displays the blood glucose concentration in mmol/l. The *BNF* lists 19 test strips and 14 proprietary meters! All of these serve the same function, and at the upper and lower ends of their calibration, all are inaccurate to within ± 20% of the true (laboratory) value. The reagent strip must be that intended for the meter.

The *BNF* advises that:

> Patients should be properly trained in the use of blood glucose monitoring systems and to take appropriate action on the results obtained. Inadequate understanding of the normal fluctuations in blood glucose may lead to

confusion and inappropriate action. It is ideal for insulin-dependent patients to observe the 'peaks' and 'troughs' of their blood glucose over 24 hours and make adjustment of their insulin dose, food intake and exercise program no more than once or twice weekly.

For type 2 diabetics who are not taking insulin, finger-prick blood glucose monitoring once weekly is usually sufficient.

Intercurrent illness

All infections stimulate the release of insulin antagonists, causing a marked rise in daily insulin requirements. If the patient becomes ill (e.g. with 'flu or community-acquired pneumonia or gastroenteritis), they should have been taught to measure the blood glucose concentration several times per day and to test the urine for ketones. Insulin-dependent diabetics should be admitted to hospital if:

- there are ketones in the urine
- there is persistent vomiting
- there is abdominal pain
- compliance is known to be poor
- the patient is a child.

Monitoring by clinicians

At every review consultation, the following tests should be done:

1 full blood count
2 full blood biochemistry, including estimated glomerular (kidney) filtration rate (eGFR) and blood urea
3 blood lipid profile
4 glycated haemoglobin (HbA_{1c}), which is a good monitor of quality of control in type 2 diabetes
5 urine testing for microalbuminuria

6 liver function tests (LFTs) for evidence of impairment, if the patient is taking a glitazone.

In addition, the following should be undertaken:

- The patient's feet should be examined for both circulation and sensation, and the patient should be referred to a podiatrist if necessary. The need for daily foot washing (avoid hot water) and general hygiene, including dental hygiene, should be stressed.
- At least once a year the patient's retinas should be examined, preferably by an eye specialist at a diabetic eye clinic.
- The patient should always be asked to keep a diary of hypoglycaemic attacks, and should always carry a few glucose tablets – these are absorbed within minutes and will abort a 'hypo reaction.'

Conclusion

After studying this chapter carefully, the student should have a good basic understanding of diabetes and its management, sufficient to enable them to appreciate what they may observe in a diabetic clinic, and to read more advanced texts with relative ease. They should also read and learn the *BNF* monographs on diabetes (Chapter 6.1). Reissued every 6 months, the *BNF* will keep the student abreast of the latest recommendations on and cautions about drug treatment.

7 Asthma

Introduction

In normal health, the lung's airways (bronchi and bronchioles) dilate during inspiration and constrict during expiration. In people with asthma there is abnormal but reversible expiratory constriction of the airways (particularly the bronchioles and smaller bronchi) in response to a variety of stimuli, depending on the individual patient. These stimuli include house dust, animal dander, seasonal pollens, respiratory infections (particularly the common cold) and exercise. Over a third of asthmatic patients have other allergic conditions, such as atopic eczema and allergic rhinitis ('hay fever'). Several common drugs precipitate asthma in asthmatic people. These include aspirin, all non-steroidal anti-inflammatory drugs (NSAIDs) and beta-adrenergic-receptor blockers. Neither the allergens nor the drugs cause wheeze in non-asthmatic people. Asthmatic wheeze is due to inflammatory cell infiltration of lung tissue, with hypertrophy of bronchiolar smooth muscle and mucus glands. This causes airway hyper-reactivity and plugging of the small airways with thick mucus.

The diagnosis of asthma must always be confirmed and the response to treatment measured by spirometry, particularly the peak expiratory flow (PEF) and the forced expiratory volume at 1 second (FEV_1). Regular recording of the PEF can be done by the patient and is very useful evidence for the therapist. It is usually lowest in the early morning and highest in the afternoon and evening.

For reasons unknown, the incidence and severity of asthma are increasing across the developed world, and asthma currently affects over 5% of the UK population. It is a chronic disorder that affects all age groups (it may first present in late middle age), but is most dangerous in children. In chronic moderate or severe asthmatics, particularly those who default on their medication (as many do), a sudden surge in bronchoconstriction may lead to an attack of acute severe asthma (formerly known as 'status asthmaticus'), which is often difficult to reverse and not infrequently fatal, accounting for 5,000 deaths and 500,000 acute hospital admissions yearly in the USA.

The three major abnormalities of asthma

These are:

1 hyper-reactivity of bronchiolar smooth muscle
2 chronic infiltration of the bronchiolar walls by inflammatory cells. Asthma is a progressive inflammatory condition in which the immune mechanisms are overactive. Understanding this central fact is essential for the doctor, the nurse and, above all, the patient
3 excessive secretion of viscid mucus which plugs the bronchioles and narrows the airways still further.

With good compliance by the patient, we are now able to treat these pathological processes effectively, because they are caused by the overactivity of chemical signals (*How Drugs Work*, Chapter 7), which modern anti-asthmatic drugs modulate or block. When studying these drug treatments, you should also learn the *BNF* guidelines (Chapter 3.1) on the management of both chronic and acute asthma in adults and children. These are revised every 6 months, and advise on the best treatments.

Non-drug treatment of asthma

Avoidance of known allergens such as house dust mite, cat dander and seasonal pollens will reduce both symptoms and underlying pathology in susceptible individuals.

Drug treatment of asthma

Table 7.1 shows the main controllers of bronchiolar tone, inflammation and mucus secretion which we target with drugs when treating asthma.

Reversing the hyper-reactivity of bronchiolar smooth muscle using selective beta$_2$-adrenergic agonists (receptor activators)

Chapters 5 and 6 of *How Drugs Work* describe receptor function using adrenoceptors as the classic example. The smooth muscle of the bronchioles is well supplied with beta$_2$-adrenoceptors, whose activation causes rapid relaxation of these muscle fibres and a consequent dilation of the air passages. We have two drugs which do this equally well – the beta$_2$-agonists salbutamol and terbutaline. These are usually taken by inhalation from a metered-dose inhaler or similar device, delivering the drug direct to the beta$_2$-receptors in the air passages. They work best when given into a spacing device, which ensures maximum drug delivery to the bronchi and bronchioles.

In mild asthma (FEV$_1$ > 80% of predicted value, with fewer than two mild episodes of wheeze per week), the beta$_2$-agonist inhaler 'when required' is the only treatment advised. Likewise, it may be all that is necessary in exercise-induced asthma – suffered by several Olympic athletes! In all other grades of asthma, the short-acting beta$_2$-agonists salbutamol and terbutaline are used as 'reliever' or 'rescue' medication to back up, as required, the regular daily medication with other drugs whose function is control of the underlying inflammation (see below).

In acute severe asthmatic episodes, much higher doses of salbutamol and terbutaline must be taken (see *BNF*, Chapter 3.1 on 'Management of severe, acute asthma in general practice'). There are two ways of achieving these large doses, and both are effective.

1 Using an inhaler spacer device to ensure better drug delivery to the bronchioles, the patient fits the metered-dose inhaler to the spacer, operates it once and inhales the air/aerosol mixture. This is repeated four to six times in quick succession. This sequence must be repeated every 10–20 minutes if necessary.

Table 7.1: The main controllers of bronchiolar tone which can be targeted when treating asthma

Bronchodilator mechanisms – actions	Drugs used	Beneficial actions in asthma
Beta$_2$-adrenoceptors on bronchial smooth muscle cause muscle relaxation, dilating the bronchioles	Beta$_2$-agonists – **short-acting:** salbutamol terbutaline	1 Cause rapid relaxation of bronchial or bronchiolar smooth muscle 2 Inhibit release of inflammatory mediation (chemical signals; see *How Drugs Work*, Chapter 5) 3 Improve clearance of mucus
	• Inhaled from metered-dose inhaler	• **The main relief/rescue medication in all grades of asthma** (see *BNF*, Chapter 3.1) Used in greatly increased dose in acute, severe asthma Few side-effects
	• Inhaled from a nebuliser	• Very high dosage – for use in severe, acute asthma with oxygen as the 'driver'
	Beta$_2$ agonists – **long-acting:** Salmeterol Formoterol	• Longer-lasting (12 hour) effects similar to salbutamol and terbutaline • To be used **only as add-on therapy** with inhaled steroids, in Stages 3, 4 and 5 (*BNF*, Chapter 3.1) • Warning: may precipitate an asthmatic attack if used alone

2 Using an oxygen-driven nebuliser, which creates an atomized spray of high-dosage salbutamol or terbutaline, 10 times the dose of an individual 'puff' from a metered-dose inhaler.

Note: In life-threatening asthma, the beta$_2$-agonist may be given by subcutaneous, intramuscular or intravenous injection.

In addition to their bronchodilating properties, the beta$_2$-agonists inhibit the release of some inflammatory chemical signals from inflammatory cells in the bronchiolar walls. They also improve the clearance of mucus. They work within 10 minutes, reach peak effect within 20–30 minutes and last for 4–6 hours.

Everyone who is treating or learning to treat asthma should learn by heart the *BNF* guidelines/protocols cited above. Patients' lives may depend on this knowledge.

Side-effects of beta$_2$-adrenoceptor agonists

Reference to *How Drugs Work*, Table 6.1 will remind you that these drugs can cause tremor, nervous tension and muscle cramps, but these side-effects are uncommon using inhaled treatment, if the inhalation technique is correct. Technique should be taught by the prescriber and checked regularly.

Longer-acting beta$_2$-agonists: a limited role in asthma prevention

In a search for improved asthmatic control, the drug industry has produced two long-acting beta$_2$-agonists, salmeterol and formoterol, with up to 12 hours' bronchodilation from a single inhaled dose, but a slow onset of action. These are currently recommended only as 'add-on' therapy for the prevention of more severe asthma (Stages 3, 4 and 5 of *BNF* guidelines, Chapter 3.1). Salmeterol and formoterol must **never** be used without an inhaled corticosteroid (see below), and patients must be warned of the possible fatal consequences if long-acting beta$_2$-agonists are used alone – an increase in the risk of severe acute asthma is associated with these drugs used alone. The reason is unclear, for they act on the same receptors as the short-acting drugs salbutamol and terbutaline. It may be safest to prescribe these long-acting beta$_2$-agonists in a combination inhaler containing, for example, fluticasone and salmeterol in fixed dose.

Controlling the inflammatory element in asthma

By regular inhalation of corticosteroids in metered doses, all the pathogenic aspects of asthma can be controlled on a long-term basis, and its progression halted and even reversed. The beneficial effects of steroids in asthma are due to their powerful damping down of inflammation and overactive immune responses. As Chapter 8 of *How Drugs Work* explains, the steroids act through steroid receptors in the bronchiolar cell nuclei, via DNA, causing synthesis of specific anti-inflammatory chemical signals which allow control of almost every aspect of asthmatic pathology (*see* Table 7.2).

- Steroids reduce both acute and chronic inflammation.
- They decrease airway hyper-reactivity/hypersensitivity.
- They stop the gradual and insidious hypertrophy (enlargement) of bronchiolar smooth muscle fibres.
- They reduce the exudate and mucus secretion which clogs the bronchioles.

The central importance of patient compliance

Effective control of all grades of asthma depends on good compliance with drug treatment, particularly regular use of the inhaled corticosteroid. Unfortunately, fewer than 40% of asthmatic patients comply adequately. The prescriber should therefore use every opportunity to urge, cajole and encourage compliance in asthmatic patients. It is always important to stress the difference between the different inhalers.

- The 'reliever/rescue' inhaler – the short-acting beta$_2$-agonists described above.
- The 'preventer' inhaler – the corticosteroids, the daily mainstay of most anti-asthmatic treatment. These will now be described.

The inhaled steroids currently available for anti-asthmatic treatment – beclometasone, budesonide, fluticasone and mometasone – are all equally effective. They must be used **regularly and continuously**, twice daily by inhalation, for all degrees of asthma except mild (see *BNF*, Chapter 3.1).

Table 7.2: Drugs used to control the bronchiolar inflammation of asthma – the preventers

	Drug	Beneficial actions in asthma
The actions of the corticosteroids (glucocorticoids)		
Steroids attenuate all aspects of the inflammatory process	**Inhaled:** beclomethasone budesonide fluticasone mometasone	Reduce acute and chronic inflammation with few side-effects Decrease airway hyper-reactivity/hypersensitivity. Stop the hypertrophy of bronchiolar smooth muscle Reduce exudate and mucus secretion Use: The regular, daily mainstay of asthma prophylaxis (prevention) in Stages 2 to 5 (see *BNF*, Chapter 3.1) Few side-effects from inhaled steroids
	Oral: prednisolone	Use: Stage 5 and acute severe asthma Risks: all steroid side-effects (see *BNF*)
The action of the immunological suppressant		
Blocks the binding of immunoglobulin IgE Mode of action in asthma is unclear Still in Phase IV of proving – intensive surveillance (*How Drugs Work*, Chapter 25)	omalizumab	In patients with proven allergic asthma and elevated serum IgE, may produce improvement as an 'add-on' therapy Specialist use only in poorly controlled asthmatics by subcutaneous injection Many very unpleasant side-effects (see *BNF*, Chapter 3.4.2)

Patients who fear the side-effects of continuous steroid medication must be repeatedly reassured that little steroid is absorbed systemically (into the bloodstream), and that side-effects are consequently slight, even in children. However, higher doses of inhaled steroids may cause adrenal suppression, and that requires specialist monitoring.

Other side-effects of inhaled steroids

The commonest is oropharyngeal thrush infection (candidiasis) due to the reduced immune response (much of all inhaled drugs is deposited on the mucous membrane of the mouth and throat). This can be greatly reduced by using a spacer device (not always convenient), by sucking antifungal lozenges or simply by rinsing the mouth and throat with water after using the inhaler.

During long-term use of higher inhaled doses of steroids, there may be some extra risk of osteoporosis in adults, and the dose of steroid should be kept at the lowest level needed to control symptoms, and titrated according to clinical response and the PEF or FEV_1 measurement. Excessive doses should be avoided in children, due to the risk of significant systemic absorption and adrenal suppression.

Oral steroids

In step 5 of the *BNF* guidelines (Chapter 3.1), oral prednisolone is added as a single daily dose. This exposes the patient to the full range of adverse steroid side-effects. Consequently, symptom-led, cautious, stepwise reduction of the oral steroid dose should be the aim. There is rarely a need to use injectable corticosteroids. As explained in *How Drugs Work*, the onset of steroid benefits is slow (12–48 hours), so the oral route is as effective as an injection, even in more severe and acute asthma.

Other anti-asthmatic drugs

Omalizumab

This is a new, immunosuppressant, third-line treatment of poorly controlled, severe asthma (*see* Table 7.2). It is mentioned for the sake of completeness – it is for specialist use only and has all the risks of immunosuppressants, but is very effective in selected patients (see *BNF*). Table 7.2 gives as much detail as the prescriber in training should need.

Leukotriene receptor blockers

Among the physiological signals that regulate the airways in normal health are bronchodilators and bronchoconstrictors. The most powerful broncho-constrictors are the leukotrienes, which cause the bronchiolar smooth muscle to contract. They also act on the bronchial mucus glands to increase mucus secretion and modulate mast-cell activity, producing inflammatory precursors. The leukotriene receptor blockers montelukast and zafirlukast (*see* Table 7.3) were developed in the expectation of a major role in blocking these effects for asthma prophylaxis. However, they are now relegated to 'add-on' treatment of Steps 3 and 4 (*BNF*, Chapter 3.1) of asthma management. (For further insight, see *How Drugs Work*, Chapter 7.)

Cholinergic-receptor blockers

Acetylcholine from the bronchiolar parasympathetic nerve fibres (vagus nerve) causes bronchoconstriction and augments mucus secretion. The cholinergic-receptor blocker ipratropium is not recommended as an asthmatic 'reliever' inhaler, but it may be given in nebulised form as an add-on treatment for life-threatening asthma (*see* Table 7.3). Along with a similar drug, tiotropium, its main use is in the long-term management of chronic obstructive pulmonary disease (COPD) (*see* Chapter 8). Due to their anticholinergic effects throughout the body, these drugs may precipitate glaucoma and prostatic bladder outflow obstruction, and cause dry mouth, nausea, constipation and occasionally tachycardia (rapid heart rate). Great care must

Table 7.3: Other main controllers of bronchiolar tone which can be targeted when treating asthma

Bronchoconstrictor mechanisms	Drugs used	Beneficial actions in asthma
Leukotriene receptors on bronchiolar smooth muscle cause intense contraction (bronchoconstriction). On the bronchiolar mucosa, leukotrienes cause increased mucus secretion	**Oral:** montelukast zafirlukast	Block leukotriene receptors, relaxing bronchiolar smooth muscle and reducing mucus secretion Many side-effects Use: As 'add-on' therapy in Stages 3 and 4
Cholinergic receptors (for parasympathetic nerves – vagus) cause bronchoconstriction and augment mucus secretion	**Inhaler or nebulizer:** ipratropium tiotropium	Block cholinergic receptors, relaxing bronchiolar smooth muscle and reducing mucus secretion For use in acute, severe and life-threatening asthma only Use: Main use is in chronic obstructive pulmonary disease (COPD), to relieve any reversible obstruction (see Chapter 8)

be taken to prevent anticholinergic spray from reaching the eyes (due to the risk of acute glaucoma).

Aminophylline

This is an old drug with limited anti-asthmatic action, some serious side-effects and many interactions with other drugs. It is occasionally given by specialists as a very slow intravenous infusion in patients with acute severe asthma. Not to be used otherwise!

Cromoglicate

This was a breakthrough in anti-asthmatic prophylaxis around 1970, effective in some patients but not in others. Its mode of action is uncertain, and it is not included in the *BNF* Management Guidelines.

Drugs which may precipitate asthma

Non-respiratory drugs which may precipitate asthma in patients with an asthmatic history (Table 7.4)

As a result of their action on one or more components of the physiological regulation of bronchiolar tone, several important and commonly used drugs can precipitate asthmatic symptoms (and indeed severe acute asthma) in patients with a history of wheeze. **It is essential that the prescriber in training knows and memorizes these, preferably by understanding why this adverse effect occurs.**

Aspirin and all non-steroidal anti-inflammatory drugs (NSAIDs)

Aspirin and all NSAIDs are potent spasmogens because they reduce the production of those prostaglandins that modulate bronchodilation by relaxing bronchiolar smooth muscle. (As explained in Chapter 7 of *How Drugs Work*, NSAIDs block the cyclo-oxygenase enzymes which catalyse prostaglandin production.) This is a most serious adverse drug reaction, and all asthmatics should be repeatedly warned to avoid aspirin and all NSAIDs. This is not a simple matter, for many proprietary preparations

Table 7.4: The main controllers of bronchiolar tone which may be blocked by systemic treatment of conditions other than asthma

Bronchodilator mechanisms affected	Blocking drugs	Adverse actions on the airways
Beta$_2$-adrenoceptors on bronchial smooth muscle serve muscle relaxation and consequent bronchodilation	**1 Cardiac – oral** Selective and non-selective beta-blockers (see *BNF*, Chapter 2.4, for list)	Block the bronchodilating beta$_2$-receptors in the bronchioles, precipitating asthma in predisposed patients
	2 Ophthalmic–topical (eye drops) Beta-blockers (see *BNF*, Chapter 11.6, for list)	Prevent access by salbutamol and terbutaline (*see* Table 7.1) to the bronchiolar beta$_2$-receptors. These are the drugs needed to relieve the asthmatic attack. If their access is blocked, they cannot work
		Therefore beta-blocking drugs should be avoided in patients with a history of asthma – as they put these individuals in double jeopardy
The prostaglandin PGE causes dilation of bronchiolar smooth muscle	Aspirin and all NSAIDs (see *BNF*, Chapter 10.1.1, for list). Many are available without prescription and widely advertised	Block the enzyme that catalyses synthesis of bronchodilating prostaglandins, including PGE
		Contraindicated in patients with a history of asthma
		Patients may not realise that they are taking an NSAID when they buy an 'over-the-counter' (OTC) medicine such as ibuprofen. Parents of asthmatic children need special warning/education about OTC medicines issued without a prescription

containing NSAIDs are freely available in pharmacies, shops and super-markets, with only 'small-print' warnings.

All beta-adrenergic blockers (selective and non-selective)

All beta-blockers may precipitate acute asthma in predisposed patients, even in minute doses (e.g. eye drops). They block the beta$_2$-receptors responsible for a large part of bronchiolar smooth muscle relaxation. Selective beta-blockers are less likely to do this, but their selectivity is relative, not absolute, and they should be avoided if possible.

One of the major problems with beta-blockers in asthmatics is that, because they block the bronchiolar beta$_2$-receptors, the latter are unresponsive to the very beta$_2$-agonist drugs, salbutamol and terbutaline, that are needed to treat the asthmatic attack. This is a major therapeutic problem.

Other asthma-precipitating drugs

Acetylcysteine (the drug used in hospital to treat paracetamol toxicity) and the dye tartrazine (an additive present in some foods) may cause acute asthma.

Conclusion

The drug treatment of asthma is one of the great success stories of modern medicine, provided that the patient complies with the regimen. Otherwise it remains an unstable condition with significant mortality and morbidity, as your experience in Accident and Emergency will testify.

8 Chronic obstructive pulmonary disease

Introduction

Chronic obstructive pulmonary disease (COPD) might be described as 'chronic lung failure.' Like chronic renal failure, it is progressive, irreversible and has more than one aetiology (cause). The disability of COPD ranges from slight dyspnoea (breathlessness) on walking to the shops or upstairs, to severe dyspnoea at rest, when the lungs are so damaged as to be unable to effect sufficient exchange of oxygen and carbon dioxide to meet the demands of the body tissues.

Around 80% of COPD is caused by smoking tobacco, and the remainder is caused by a variety of industrial dusts and other pollutants. Other factors may be involved, e.g. genetic predisposition, since only about 15% of lifelong smokers develop COPD. Progression of COPD often ceases after stopping smoking.

Many COPD patients have features of both chronic bronchitis and emphysema, differentiated by symptoms, spirometry (essential for establishing the severity of COPD), and in severe cases, blood and blood-gas analysis. In both chronic bronchitis and emphysema there is progressive obstruction of airflow, loss of respiratory gas-exchange capacity and progressively disabling dyspnoea. Where the inflammation of chronic bronchitis predominates, there is also chronic cough and mucopurulent sputum, both made worse by any respiratory infection. In emphysema the problem is progressive destruction of the gas-exchange surfaces of the lungs (the alveoli), and there may be little cough or sputum.

A proportion of COPD patients have bronchial hyper-reactivity which is sometimes reversible using bronchodilator inhalers like those used in asthma, but many patients show no such response. All COPD patients should be tested for reversible bronchoconstriction because, if present, its treatment gives substantial improvement of symptoms.

Prescribers should always remind themselves of the aims of their interventions. In the case of COPD, the main aims are:

1 relief of the symptoms of breathlessness, cough and sputum

2 improvement of exercise capacity and reduction of restrictions in lifestyle

3 prevention of acute deteriorations (exacerbations), and prompt treatment when they occur

4 slowing of disease progression (unlike asthma, it cannot be prevented)

5 minimizing hospitalizations and extending lifespan.

These aims will not be achieved unless both the non-drug and drug treatments are enthusiastically applied by the patient as well as by the professionals and carers. So the non-drug treatments must be part of your 'prescription' from the start (i.e. your management plan).

Non-drug treatment of COPD

Smoking cessation is the only effective treatment to improve future quality of life and reduce disability and death. Thereafter, a combination of smoking cessation, cough training (to improve the discharge of mucopus) and other respiratory physiotherapy, including graded exercise regimens, are essential daily treatment for all COPD patients. For the more severe cases, the addition of continuous oxygen supplementation improves patients' quality of life, reduces hospitalizations and extends lifespan. Flu vaccination in autumn and spring is important. Polyvalent pneumococcal vaccine, repeated every 6 years, is advocated by some authorities. Where it is available, pulmonary rehabilitation improves quality of life and reduces readmissions to hospital.

Drug treatment of COPD

When considering drug treatment of COPD, one must realize that only a limited improvement may be achieved. However, in severe COPD, even a 20% improvement in respiratory function may greatly improve the patient's quality of life (and that of his or her family).

Bronchodilator inhalers/nebulizers

Anticholinergic bronchodilators

Ipratropium bromide gives valuable relief of dyspnoea and wheeze in those patients who have a reversible element of airway restriction. It blocks the cholinergic receptors in the bronchi and bronchioles which stimulate bronchoconstriction (*see* Chapter 7 for more detail). Ipratropium should be inhaled up to four times daily, in doses graded to the patient's response.

Tiotropium inhaled once daily has a similar action but a faster onset and longer duration of action.

Either of these drugs should be used regularly, in the dose and frequency that the patient requires. COPD is their primary licensed use ('indication'), and they should not be used 'as required.'

Beta$_2$-adrenoceptor-agonist bronchodilators

In COPD with a reversible element of airway restriction, salbutamol or terbutaline are as effective in relieving dyspnoea as the anticholinergic agents just described. They stimulate the beta$_2$-adrenoceptors on bronchial and bronchiolar smooth muscle, which causes relaxation of the smooth muscle and consequent dilation of the airways (see *How Drugs Work*, Chapters 5 and 6).

Choosing the most appropriate bronchodilator in COPD

There are many 'guidelines', but the *BNF* is among the most helpful (see *BNF*, Chapter 3.1 on 'Chronic obstructive pulmonary disease'), and the following is an adaptation of this guidance.

1 In mild COPD, occasional use of the beta$_2$-agonist inhalers salbutamol or

terbutaline (together with all the non-drug treatments above) may be all that is needed.

2 In moderate and severe airway obstruction, **regular** use of the anticholinergic inhalers ipratropium or tiotropium should be added to the inhaled salbutamol or terbutaline.

3 It is usual to give newly presenting COPD patients a trial course of high-dose inhaled corticosteroid, for up to 12 weeks, monitoring spirometry results. If the patient's forced expiratory volume at 1 second (FEV_1) has not increased by more than 20%, the steroid should be stopped. Beclometasone, fluticasone and budesonide are equally effective.

4 In severe COPD (FEV_1 less than 50% of predicted value), a trial of high-dose inhaled or oral corticosteroid, combined on specialist recommendation with a long-acting beta$_2$-agonist inhaler should be given, but this should be discontinued if there is no improvement after 4 weeks. (For more detail on the action of these drugs, *see* Chapter 7.)

Caution: There is now clear evidence that the long-acting beta$_2$-agonists formoterol and salmeterol should not be used alone, but always in combination with a corticosteroid inhaler or tablet. They may precipitate severe wheeze, if used alone.

5 Long-term continuous oxygen should be given to all patients with severe COPD, usually via nasal tubes ('spectacles'). It has no ill effects, relieves symptoms, improves mobility and quality of life, reduces hospitalizations and extends life. Oxygen concentrator pumps are supplied to the patient's home. (See the excellent section on oxygen in the *BNF*, Chapter 3.6.)

6 In all COPD treatment, assess the response by improvement (or lack of it) in symptoms as well as spirometry. Always use symptoms and spirometry to individualize your treatment regimens. The FEV_1 and the forced vital capacity (FVC) are both required, and the FEV_1:FVC ratio is often used to quantify progress.

Treating acute episodes of COPD (exacerbations)

Especially during the winter months and during infection with a cold or 'flu, the dyspnoea, cough and sputum of COPD often increase. These exacerbations are much worse when acute bronchitis occurs. Acute bronchitis may initially be viral in origin, but secondary bacterial infection is usual, involving several pathogenic bacterial species. In this situation, broad-spectrum antibiotics are usually added to the patient's treatment regimen (which may need increased bronchodilator dosages). Co-amoxyclav or doxycycline are the usual 'menu' in the community, given in high oral dosage for at least 10 days.

Do not expect a dramatic response, for many pathogenic bacteria in the community are resistant to several antibiotics (multi-drug resistance). In a given patient, a proportion of these bacteria will be resistant, and giving an antibiotic is likely to clear competing 'normal' bacterial flora from the lungs and allow the resistant organisms to proliferate and colonize the lungs. This may leave the patient in a worse state than if no antibiotic had been given (see *How Drugs Work*, Chapter 22).

Antibiotics should probably be reserved for severe COPD exacerbations. In hospital, they would always be given in conjunction with nebulized bronchodilators, oral corticosteroids and continuous oxygen.

Remember that COPD deterioration can be due to the development of lung cancer, overuse of sedatives (reducing airflow) or pneumothorax (air entering the pleural cavity between the lung and the chest wall).

When to admit a COPD patient to hospital

Urgent hospital admission is essential if:

1 there is a sudden increase in symptom severity, particularly breathlessness to the point of distress (indicating a poor response to treatment)
2 cyanosis occurs (lips and fingers turn purple-blue in colour). It indicates severe hypoxia (insufficient oxygen to saturate the haemoglobin in the red blood cells)

3 if, in addition, the patient is elderly, or has heart failure, diabetes or any other chronic condition.

Theophylline/aminophylline

These are very risky drugs with limited efficacy. Their use is the preserve of respiratory specialists.

Cough medicines

These are all of placebo value only, but this may be helpful to a patient with severe COPD.

Conclusion

Read the paragraph on non-drug treatment again – it is the mainstay of good COPD management.

9 Community-acquired pneumonia

Introduction

Community-acquired pneumonia (CAP) is a common, serious disease of the lower respiratory tract, in which the lung tissues are colonized (invaded) by one of a range of pathogens (disease-causing micro-organisms), from viruses to several types of bacteria, most notably the pneumococcus (*Streptococcus pneumoniae*), *Haemophilus influenzae*, *Chlamydia*, *Mycoplasma* and *Legionella*. CAP often follows an acute upper respiratory tract infection (URTI), and is characterized by the acute or subacute onset of fever, dyspnoea (breathlessness) and cough. There may be abnormal breath sounds on auscultation (stethoscope examination). Sweating and shivering are common, as is chest discomfort. The patient feels ill and tired, and looks it. As the condition progresses, there may be haemoptysis (coughing blood or bloodstained phlegm) and an increased respiratory rate, a rapid pulse and a marked decrease in both systolic and diastolic blood pressure. Pleurisy (inflammation of the lungs' covering membrane) may occur, causing sharp, localized chest pain on deep breathing and coughing.

Death results from CAP in around 1% of cases, rising to over 10% in the elderly and those with chronic heart failure, renal failure, liver failure, a deficient immune system or cancer. (CAP patients who require hospital admission sustain over 20% mortality.) This risk of death is reduced by prompt diagnosis and treatment.

How does CAP differ from hospital-acquired pneumonia?

CAP is pneumonia that begins to develop outside hospital in patients who have not been inpatients. The invading organisms are often found among the normal flora of the human upper respiratory tract. Hospital-acquired pneumonia (HAP) occurs after admission to hospital for some other serious condition. It is caused by a variety of often antibiotic-resistant bacteria from a number of sources, most commonly intensive-care units (ICUs) in patients who are being mechanically ventilated. HAP is the main cause of death due to hospital-acquired infection (over 20% mortality), and it presents very difficult treatment problems for medical microbiologists. Its treatment is specialized and need not be described here.

Nursing-home-acquired pneumonia

Apart from the fact that patients in nursing homes are often frail and elderly, there is some evidence that when they develop pneumonia, the causative bacteria are generally similar to those that cause CAP. Consequently, similar treatment regimens should be used (see below). Due to their age (> 65 years) they are more likely to require hospital admission.

Assess the patient before treating CAP – using CRB65

CRB65 is a well-established mnemonic that uses only the clinical evidence available to the doctor or nurse in the community, allowing immediate assessment and reassessment of the severity of CAP. Each clinical sign contributes a single point, and the total score (from 0 to 5) is applied to Figure 9.1, to determine the proper course of action. The clinical signs C, R, B and 65 are as follows:

- Confusion in a previously unconfused patient (or increasing confusion in a previous slightly confused patient).

- Respiratory rate ≥ 30/minute (normal value *c.* 12/minute).
- Blood pressure < 90 mmHg systolic or < 60 mmHg diastolic.
- 65 years or older.

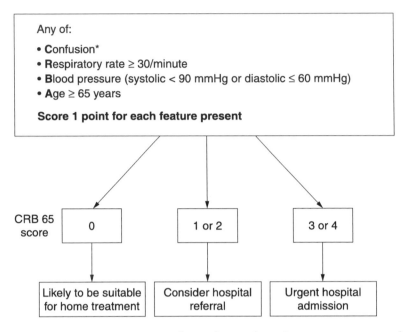

Figure 9.1: Severity assessment used to determine the management of CAP in patients in the community (CRB65 score), updated in 2004. British Thoracic Society Guidelines (2004). *Defined as a Mental Test Score of 8 or less, or new disorientation in respect of person, place or time.

As Figure 9.1 shows, a total score of 1 or above merits urgent hospital admission, or at least a consultant physician's opinion, since it is associated with a fivefold increased risk of death.

If a blood urea measurement is available, a value above 7 mmol/l contributes a further predictive point (U), converting CRB65 to the hospital mnemonic of CURB65, but CRB65 is quite adequate for community assessment of CAP. The blood urea concentration should certainly be included in a twice-daily reassessment of CURB65, if you opt for community treatment.

All children suspected of having pneumonia must be admitted without delay to a specialized paediatric intensive-care unit.

Treatment of CAP

General measures

1   A sputum sample and two pre-antibiotic blood cultures should be taken for bacteriology. Do not delay specific treatment by waiting for results (see section on specific treatment below).

2   A full blood count and serum electrolytes and urea should be sent for urgent analysis.

3   A pulse oximeter should be used to estimate the patient's haemoglobin oxygen saturation. This fits like a single-finger glove on the patient's index finger. Supplementary oxygen should be available from a concentrator, via nasal 'spectacles.'

4   Near-patient screening for the causative organisms should soon be generally available, based on the presence of urinary antigens to specific organisms – pneumococcus and *Legionella*.

5   The patient must stop smoking, stay in bed and drink copious fluids.

6   Analgesia (pain relief) is important if the patient develops pleurisy, e.g. strong co-codamol tablets (30/500) in the dose needed to relieve the pain, with senna tablets to prevent the severe constipation that results from codeine. Stronger opioids (morphine-like drugs) are not recommended, since they all depress the respiratory control mechanisms.

Specific treatment: which antibiotic?

(Revise Chapter 22, on antibiotic action and bacterial resistance, in *How Drugs Work.*)

Ideally, all antibiotic treatment should be based on the results of bacteriology (knowledge of the causative organism and its antibiotic sensitivity). That takes up to 48 hours from sampling, and this delay could prove fatal in CAP. Therefore it is accepted practice to prescribe an antibiotic 'empirically' (a euphemism for prescribing blindly) as soon as the diagnosis is firm.

The *BNF* (Chapter 5) offers the community prescriber the choice of:

1 amoxycillin orally, 500 mg to 1 g every 8 hours for 7 days, or (if the patient is penicillin-allergic)

2 clarithromycin orally, 250–500 mg every 12 hours for 7 days.

Whichever antibiotic is chosen to treat CAP, it is vital to give it in high doses, typically double or more of the dose advised for less severe infections. The reason is that some common pathogenic bacteria in CAP have what is called 'low-level' or 'relative' antibiotic resistance – they are resistant to standard doses of antibiotic but sensitive to sustained higher doses. Chapter 22 in *How Drugs Work* emphasizes the need to sustain antibiotic concentrations by precise timing of doses. You should also request regular (e.g. 6-monthly) data from your area microbiology laboratory on the pattern of antibiotic resistance in the common community bacterial pathogens, together with the laboratory's recommendations as to 'best-guess' antibiotics for different infections. Currently, up to 5% (and 35% in parts of the USA) of community pneumococci isolated in the laboratory are resistant to amoxycillin, and 15% are resistant to erythromycin. You should suspect this if a patient fails to respond to treatment, and refer them at once for specialized advice.

Pneumonia is prone to cause complications in 5–20% of patients. These may involve the lungs (pleural effusion or empyema – pus in the pleural space), heart (cardiac failure or infections), brain (meningitis) and other organs. Descriptions of these serious sequelae are beyond the scope of this introductory book. Details will be found in a more advanced text.

This emphasizes the need for at least twice daily review of a patient with CAP, whether at home or in a nursing home. Reassess the patient's chest and general condition using CURB65, and admit them to hospital if there is either deterioration or an inadequate response to treatment.

Finally, remember that lung cancer can present as pneumonia, often with relatively few signs on examination.

10 Dyspepsia (upper gastrointestinal symptoms)

Introduction

Symptoms originating in the gastrointestinal tract (GIT) (oesophagus, stomach, small intestine and colon) are often vague, misleading and unreliable for the purpose of reaching a diagnosis. No firm diagnosis should be made on the basis of gastrointestinal symptoms alone. Neither should any medium- or long-term treatment be based on symptoms. Indeed, serious disease of the GIT is completely asymptomatic in some patients, while in others, intensive investigation of unpleasant chronic symptoms not infrequently fails to identify any GIT pathology.

So when a patient presents with one or other form of dyspepsia ('indigestion', 'heartburn', 'stomach ache', etc.), it is important to remember that it may be a simple self-limiting problem, or one that requires long-term management with powerful modern drugs, or rarely, the first symptom of a cancer of the upper GIT.

The importance of history-taking in dyspeptic patients

A thorough history should be taken from the patient – it need take only 2 or 3 minutes. The following checklist gives the basic minimal history you must elicit.

1 What exactly are the symptoms?

2 How long have they been present?

3 How severe are the symptoms?

4 When do they occur during the 24-hour day (e.g. are they worse at night)?

5 Where are they felt?

6 What brings them on (e.g. a meal or lying flat)?

7 What relieves the symptoms?

8 What medicines are being taken for any condition(s), including herbal and over-the-counter medicines?

Above all, ask specifically about the 'ALARM' symptoms. These may indicate a cancer of the stomach or oesophagus or an ulcer that is about to haemorrhage or perforate, needing urgent referral to a gastroenterologist, so it is important to exclude them as routine.

1 Is there persistent vomiting?

2 Has the patient vomited blood or dark brown 'coffee-grounds' material (blood altered by gastric acid), even once?

3 Is there difficulty in swallowing, especially food sticking on the way down (dysphagia)?

4 Has the patient been losing weight (unintentionally)?

5 Has the patient passed any very dark stools, even once?

6 Is the patient over 50 years old?

If there is an upper abdominal mass on examination and/or anaemia on blood testing, the likelihood of serious pathology is even greater.

If the 'ALARM' symptoms are absent, it is usual to divide symptoms into two groups:

1 reflux-like symptoms

2 ulcer-like symptoms.

Note that there may be overlap and, as noted above, GIT symptoms are not well localized in some patients.

Reflux-like symptoms lasting more than a few weeks

The term 'reflux' refers to gastric acid entering the oesophagus, and is short for 'gastro-oesophageal reflux.'

Reflux-like symptoms include:

* 'heartburn' – discomfort or pain radiating from the stomach area into the throat
* 'waterbrash' – acidic phlegm in the throat
* 'regurgitation' – bringing stomach contents into the mouth.

These symptoms are often worse following a meal or on lying down, and are usually relieved by taking an antacid. One or more of them is often (but not always) present in gastro-oesophageal reflux disease (GORD).

Ulcer-like symptoms lasting more than a few weeks

* Well localized pain in the epigastrium (centre of upper abdomen).
* Often worse at night.
* Often relieved by meals and/or antacids. Remember to ask the patient about medicines from the pharmacist, which may now include powerful acid suppressants such as proton pump inhibitors (see *How Drugs Work*, Chapter 8) and histamine H_2-blockers (see *How Drugs Work*, Chapter 6).
* Patient is often a heavy smoker.
* On examination, there is often tenderness on deep palpation of the epigastrium.

You will discover on history-taking of GIT symptoms that there are several vague symptoms which may be very real to the patient, but which are unlikely to be related either to reflux disease (GORD) or to peptic ulcer disease. These symptoms include:

* bloating – distension of abdomen after a meal
* flatulence
* vague nausea
* poorly localized pain – no tenderness on palpation.

Finally (with regard to history taking), you must learn the list of commonly used drugs which may all cause dyspepsia, and you must find out whether the patient is taking any of them (usually as part of a long-term medication regimen). Drugs that may cause dyspepsia include:

1 NSAIDs – non-steroidal anti-inflammatory drugs are the commonest cause of peptic ulceration

2 nitrates – anti-anginal medicines

3 oral steroids – synthetic glucocorticoids for chronic severe inflammation

4 bisphosphonates – for osteoporosis

5 theophylline/aminophylline – sometimes still used for poorly controlled asthma and chronic obstructive pulmonary disease (COPD) (under consultant guidance)

6 calcium-channel blockers for hypertension and other heart problems.

Note that patients often do not know the name(s) of their drug(s), and it may be necessary to get a treatment summary, or ask the patient to bring all their medications to you.

In summary, although upper GIT presenting symptoms are often vague, careful history taking will usually 'sharpen' the evidence, sometimes sufficiently to allow definitive treatment. The clinician in training should cultivate a high index of suspicion – if you don't, you will miss the 1–5% of serious illness that requires full specialist investigation.

Treating dyspepsia

Presumptive treatment (without further investigation)

Such is the frequency of dyspeptic symptoms in primary care that it is unrealistic to send all such patients for specialist investigations such as oesphagoscopy and gastroscopy. Indeed, 60% of the limited number of patients who are referred for 'scoping' have no identifiable pathology and are classified as having 'functional dyspepsia.' Recognizing this, the current National Institute for Health and Clinical Excellence (NICE) guidelines in the UK give the following advice.

1 Stop dyspepsia-causing drugs, if this is possible (often not).

2 Give robust advice about the patient's lifestyle, namely:

- stop smoking

- reduce intake of fatty foods

- lose weight

- use antacids with alginate (the alkali neutralizes the gastric hydrochloric acid and the alginate forms a protective coating along the oesophagus and a protective raft above the stomach acid).

3 Review the patient after 1 month.

4 If at this review there is an inadequate response (i.e. symptoms are not much improved), prescribe a proton pump inhibitor (PPI) in full dose, e.g. omeprazole or lansoprazole.

PPIs are the ultimate gastric acid suppressants. Chapter 8 of *How Drugs Work* describes their action, which is to block the carrier mechanism in the gastric acid-secreting (parietal) cells, preventing the secretion of H^+ ions into the gastric lumen (the stomach cavity).

Caveat regarding the NICE guideline to prescribe PPIs 'blind' (presumptively)

This NICE recommendation to prescribe a powerful PPI acid suppressant presumptively in full dosage is a pragmatic compromise of best practice, which is ideally never to use any powerful modern drug unless a 'definite' or 'very probable' diagnosis has been made. In the case of full-dose PPIs, the particular reason for caution is that PPIs will temporarily heal not only benign peptic ulcers, but also gastric mucosa ulcerated by a pre-malignant or malignant growth. The prescriber should keep this in mind if the patient returns with a recurrence of symptoms. Suspicion and an alert and informed mind are the hallmarks of a good clinician.

The next stage: a definitive diagnosis

Referral to a gastroenterologist will often result in oesophago-gastroscopy, a procedure that involves inserting a flexible tube with a light, a fibre-optic scope and a biopsy clip down the oesophagus, which is then examined throughout its length. The entire stomach and duodenal antrum are then inspected. Biopsies are taken of any suspicious areas. The possible findings are as follows:

- normal tissues throughout – a valuable, reassuring result
- an abnormality in the oesophagus:
  - chronic inflammatory changes due to long-term reflux of gastric acid
  - Barrett's oesophagus, also due to chronic acid reflux, in which condition the normal oesophageal lining mucosa has been replaced by mucous membrane similar in structure to that of the stomach or duodenum. Barrett's oesophagus is a pre-cancerous condition that requires regular scoping – a proportion of these patients will develop oesophageal cancer
  - a hiatus hernia, where a section of upper stomach has herniated (pushed through) the diaphragm
  - evidence of oesophageal cancer, proven on biopsy
- an abnormality of the stomach or duodenum:
  - varying degrees of erosive gastritis (damage to stomach mucosa by its own acid)
  - benign ulceration of the stomach or duodenum (a peptic ulcer)
  - a gastric cancer
  - atrophic gastritis (a marked thinning of the mucosa, often associated with pernicious anaemia).

  A firm diagnosis allows logical specific drug treatment as follows.

Treatment of chronic gastro-oesophageal reflux disease (GORD), including Barrett's oesophagus and hiatus hernia

1 The general measures prescribed by NICE (*see* above).

2 A proton pump inhibitor (PPI). It is customary to use this in high dosage (i.e. until symptoms have cleared completely – usually 1 to 2 months) and then to keep most patients on a lower maintenance dose. The reason is that GORD represents a failure of the body's anti-reflux mechanism (the gastro-oesophageal sphincter), and relapse often occurs if the PPI is

stopped. No serious long-term effects have been found on chronic PPI use, although the *BNF* records a considerable list of side-effects (*BNF*, Chapter 1.3.5), and PPIs interact with several other drugs, including warfarin (see *BNF*, Appendix 1 and *How Drugs Work*, Chapter 23). The maintenance dose of PPI is often the only treatment that is needed.

There is a common misconception (unfortunately implicit in the NICE guidelines) that eradication of the bacterium *Helicobacter pylori* from the stomach is advisable when treating GORD. There is no evidence that *Helicobacter pylori* causes or worsens GORD, and this bacterium colonizes a large proportion of healthy people with no known ill effects. *Helicobacter pylori* eradication therapy (see below) should be reserved for proven or probable peptic ulcer disease (and such treatment has several unpleasant and some serious side-effects) rather than used routinely for GORD.

If the symptoms of GORD and hiatus hernia cannot be controlled using long-term PPI treatment, surgery may be considered in order to tighten the gastro-oesophageal sphincter (fundoplication). However, this procedure is not without risk, complications and, within a few years, failure of the fundoplication with recurrence of the GORD symptoms.

Treatment of benign peptic ulcer

Over 90% of gastric ulcers and duodenal ulcers are associated with *Helicobacter pylori* colonization of the stomach, and eradication of *Helicobacter pylori* is curative in the large majority of these ulcers. Moreover, the cure is often permanent. The presence of *Helicobacter pylori* can be proved non-invasively in the primary care setting using the urea breath test (instructions come with the test, but see a more advanced text for details). For breath testing, the patient should be off PPI medication for 2 weeks. There are several equally good treatment regimens (see *BNF*, Chapter 1.3), e.g. a combination of:

> amoxycillin 500 mg, thrice daily
> metronidazole 500 mg, thrice daily   } for 1 week.
> omeprazole 20 mg, twice daily

Caveat on national guidelines (e.g. NICE)

The guideline recommendation to apply a *Helicobacter pylori* eradication regimen 'blind' (before positive diagnosis or even proof of the presence of *Helicobacter pylori*) is another compromise of ideal practice. It subjects those patients who do not have peptic ulceration to the unnecessary side-effects and risks of the regimen, some of which are serious, including the risk of the sometimes fatal antibiotic-associated colitis (due to *Clostridium difficile*).

11 Vomiting, diarrhoea and constipation

Introduction

Vomiting and diarrhoea of acute (sudden) onset, lasting 24–48 hours, without fever, are **not diseases**, but symptoms indicating that the body is expelling toxic or infected material from the intestine, and clearing the intestine of the substrate on which bacteria feed.

A variety of micro-organisms cause gastroenteritis, including the *Salmonella* group of bacteria (typhoid and paratyphoid), *Shigella* (dysentery), *Campylobacter* species, *Clostridium* species, *Escherichia coli* type 0157:H7 and *Staphylococcus aureus* (via toxins in infected food). Several enteroviruses cause epidemics of gastroenteritis in crowded communities (e.g. cruise ships, army barracks, prisons, etc.), particularly the rotavirus and norovirus. Several protozoans (amoeba-like organisms) are common pathogens, e.g. *Giardia*, *Cryptosporidium* and *Entamoeba*.

All of these infections are spread by poor food hygiene and personal hygiene, and are transmitted from person to person by infected food, water and hands.

All antibiotics can cause diarrhoea by disrupting the normal colonic bacterial flora. Rarely in the community, but sometimes fatally, toxic antibiotic-associated colitis (due to *Clostridium difficile*) follows. This is a major emergency which should be suspected if diarrhoea occurs within 3 weeks of a course of oral antibiotics. Antibiotic-resistant *C. diff.* infections are now common in many hospitals, and often fatal.

Treatment of acute vomiting and diarrhoea

In most cases, the only treatment needed is rest and plentiful fluid replacement, especially in children. Balanced electrolyte preparations include Dioralyte, Rapolyte and Electrolade, made up as directed in clean drinking water (or boiled water if the available water is suspect). The vomiting and diarrhoea are part of the body's curative response to the infection. Although anti-motility drugs like codeine phosphate, cophenotrope and loperamide are popular and widely advertised, it is usually better to avoid using them, since they reduce the diarrhoea at the expense of retaining the billions of infecting organisms and their toxins, which the diarrhoea would have expelled. All of the drugs are opioids (morphine-like), and all of them act on the opioid N and S receptors in the nerve plexuses of the gut wall (*see How Drugs Work*, Chapter 14). Cophenotrope also contains atropine.

Anti-emetics like prochlorperazine can give short-term relief of vomiting. It is one of several dopamine-receptor blockers that act on the chemoreceptor trigger zone (CTZ) of the brainstem, which is part of the vomiting control mechanism (*see How Drugs Work*, Chapter 15). A more powerful anti-emetic is metoclopramide, which acts as a dopamine antagonist (receptor blocker) in the CTZ, and locally in the stomach and intestine, promoting increased peristalsis and consequent movement of stomach and intestinal contents by acting as an agonist (stimulant) of the serotonin $5HT_4$ receptors in the intestinal wall (*see How Drugs Work*, Chapter 15), a so-called 'prokinetic' function. *See BNF*, Chapter 4.6 for side-effects.

The most powerful anti-emetic drugs, used to control the intense nausea of cancer chemotherapy, are the 'setrons', e.g. granisetron. A discussion of their use is beyond the scope of this book (*see How Drugs Work*, Chapter 15).

If vomiting or diarrhoea becomes worse, persists beyond 48 hours or is accompanied by a high fever (> 39°C/101°F), you must suspect that the infection has spread into the intestinal wall and beyond (systemic spread). Stool samples should be sent for bacteriology/virology and the patient transferred urgently to hospital, particularly in the case of a child. The presence of abdominal pain and tenderness or blood in the stools are warnings that require hospitalization. The elderly and AIDs sufferers are particularly at risk.

Note that the strain of *E. coli* 0157:H7 produces toxins which are particularly risky in young children, who are in any case most at risk of dehydration and plasma electrolyte imbalance due to the diarrhoea and vomiting.

Likewise, bloodstained vomit (or 'coffee-grounds' vomit – blood altered by gastric acid) and bloody diarrhoea are both indications for immediate hospital admission. Black stools (melaena) indicate significant bleeding from the stomach or small intestine, and are a surgical emergency.

Chronic diarrhoea (> 4–6 weeks) requires referral to a specialist for investigation. It may be a symptom of inflammatory bowel disease (ulcerative colitis or Crohn's disease), malabsorption, malignancy or gastrointestinal parasitic infestation. These are serious diseases with marked morbidity and significant mortality, often resistant to treatment, particularly if diagnosis is delayed.

Constipation

'Constipation' is one of the vaguest symptoms, and needs careful history-taking to explore what the patient is actually experiencing. The patient may mean infrequent stools, hard stools, straining or pain on defecation, or a feeling of incomplete evacuation. 'Normal' bowel function ranges from two soft stools per day to one large, firm stool every third day. So the individual will relate the term 'constipation' to their 'normal' or 'regular' habit. The commonest causes are:

- inadequate dietary fibre
- enforced inactivity (e.g. elderly patients and those in hospital)
- many commonly used drugs (*see* Table 11.1).

Constipation is often a feature of hypothyroidism, a frequently missed diagnosis, easily revealed by a thyroid function test (TFT) on a venous blood sample and is easily and fully treatable.

Table 11.1: Some drugs that cause constipation

Codeine in the analgesic co-codamol
Morphine and all the related opioids
Tricyclic antidepressants
The calcium-channel blocker verapamil
Chronic laxative use/abuse
Lithium
Iron
Some antacids (calcium carbonate or aluminium hydroxide)
Anti-parkinsonian drugs of the anticholinergic type (e.g. benzotropine,
  orphenadrine)
Anti-diarrhoeal drugs (see above)
The phenothiazines (an anti-psychotic drug group)

Treatment of the symptoms of constipation

1 Increase the patient's intake of fluids and fibre (e.g. by adding bran in any form).

2 Encourage activity – abdominal exercises that can be performed in bed are effective and easily taught.

3 Minimise constipating drugs.

4 Supplement the dietary fibre if necessary, using methylcellulose or ispaghula husk (these increase faecal bulk and retain water, softening the stool).

5 Oral stimulant laxatives should be used only occasionally. The mildest is the herbal derivative senna, and the strongest is sodium picosulphate.

6 Liquid paraffin oral emulsion BP is an effective faecal softener, but the *BNF* specifies 'Avoid prolonged use', due to a range of side-effects (see *BNF*, Chapter 1.6.3).

7 Dantron is a powerful stimulant laxative reserved for constipation in terminal illness. It is carcinogenic (may cause cancer), and often causes excoriation of the perianal skin.

8 Stimulant enemas are reserved for severe constipation in elderly and bedbound patients, and before X-ray studies of the colon, e.g. phosphate enema BPC.

9 Non-absorbable fluids such as the macrogols (see *BNF*) or osmotic agents such as lactulose are used to supplement increased fluid and fibre intake.

Remember the 'ALARM' signals in both chronic diarrhoea and constipation

The following, particularly if two or more are present, should alert you to the fact that serious underlying pathology is present, e.g. colorectal cancer or inflammatory bowel disease:

1 a change in bowel habit to looser stools and/or increased frequency, lasting more than 6 weeks

2 rectal bleeding (excluding bleeding piles)

3 iron-deficiency anaemia, particularly if the haemoglobin concentration is < 8 g/dl

4 a palpable mass in the abdomen or rectum.

Note that constipation is not often due to colorectal cancer, unless the intestinal lumen has been obstructed by the tumour.

Irritable bowel syndrome (IBS)

This is not an easy diagnosis to make in primary care. A variety of chronic symptoms may present, including variable and varying abdominal pain, usually poorly localised, a sense of bloating, diarrhoea, constipation or a sense of incomplete defecation. A gastroenterologist might consider IBS as a diagnosis in the proven absence of structural, medical or neurological disease. A recent international consensus on symptoms typical of IBS (the Rome II Criteria) may be found helpful:

> The presence for at least 12 weeks (which need not be consecutive) in the preceding 12 months of abdominal discomfort or pain that has two of the following three features:

- relieved with defaecation
- onset associated with a change in the frequency of stool
- onset associated with a change in form (appearance) of stool.

There is no specific treatment, and a variety of treatments may be tried with the aim of relieving the symptoms rather than curing them. For example:

- increased dietary fibre (may worsen IBS!)
- anti-motility drugs such as loperamide to lessen diarrhoea
- anti-spasmodic drugs such as mebeverine to relieve colic
- a tricyclic antidepressant in low dosage, for its anticholinergic effect on the intestinal neurons, lessening colicky, poorly coordinated peristalsis
- an exclusion diet (administered by a dietitian), which sometimes reveals a link between IBS symptoms and particular foods.

12 Arthritis

Joint pain and stiffness account for about 15% of all primary care consultations, and are by far the largest causes of physical disability (*c*. 35% of all causes). 'Arthritis' and 'rheumatism' are complex specialist subjects, so this chapter will give only an introduction to the two commonest forms of joint disease, namely osteoarthritis (OA) and rheumatoid arthritis (RA).

Introduction

The normal limb joints

The limb joints are among the wonders of human structure and function. Think of their ranges of movement, weight-bearing capacity and tolerance of shear and stress over a lifetime of up to a century. What is not so obvious is the way in which intra-articular friction has been reduced to that of ice on ice! The articulating ends of each limb bone are covered with a layer of articular cartilage which is ultra-low-friction, wear-resistant, elastic and slightly compressible. The rest of the joint is encased by the synovial membrane, which secretes the synovial fluid that is involved in the nutrition, lubrication and protection from erosion of the articular cartilages. So robust are the joints that many people reach old age without joint pain or loss of function. However, in both osteoarthritis and rheumatoid arthritis there is a breakdown of normal joint structure and function, with progressive loss of function, pain and stiffness.

Osteoarthritis (OA)

OA is due mainly to life's wear and tear – it is degenerative joint disease and so is commonest in older people. Slow degeneration of the articular cartilage is accompanied by hypertrophy (overgrowth) of bone at its margin. In OA there is often little inflammation. OA is more common in joints which have been injured in the past or regularly over-stressed, e.g. the hips and knees of obese people and those with abnormal posture or gait.

OA symptoms usually begin with short-lived morning stiffness, but patients generally seek help only when this later develops into pain on movement, that is relieved by rest. On examination, the range of passive movement may be normal until later in the process. The only physical finding may be a grating, creaking sensation (crepitus) under the examining fingers when the joint is moved. The joint is **seldom** swollen with fluid or warm to the touch.

Treating osteoarthritis

OA cannot be cured or its progress much slowed by any drugs. The aim is to maintain function and relieve pain. The nature of pain, its nerve pathways and the actions of analgesic drugs (pain-relievers) are explained in *How Drugs Work*, Chapter 14. Pain relief in OA should begin with oral paracetamol, raising the dose as required to 1 gram, four times daily. Codeine phosphate 30 mg, four times daily, may be added when paracetamol alone gives inadequate relief. The most troublesome side-effect of this drug is constipation, and laxatives are sometimes needed. The combination of paracetamol 500 mg and codeine phosphate 30 mg (co-codamol 30/500) is often prescribed. Always remember that about 10% of each dose of codeine is metabolized to morphine, and that long-term use of co-codamol may cause dependence and tolerance (see *How Drugs Work*, Chapter 19).

On the 'analgesic staircase', the next step is to opiates (morphine and related drugs, including tramadol), with the full range of opioid side-effects (see *BNF*, Chapter 4.7.2). There are no 'intermediate' analgesics at present.

Since there is usually little joint inflammation in OA, the use of non-steroidal anti-inflammatory drugs (NSAIDs) such as ibuprofen or diclofenac is illogical. They have no effect on the joint damage, and their analgesic effect is no better than the plain analgesics just described. Above all, NSAIDs have a devastating list of serious adverse effects, including damage to the stomach and kidneys, worsening of hypertension (raised blood pressure), congestive heart failure, asthma, exacerbation of inflammatory bowel disease and psoriasis (see *How Drugs Work*, Chapter 7). Over 30% of all reported adverse drug events are due to NSAIDs! Despite this, they are often prescribed in primary care. If they are used at all, only those NSAIDs with the lowest incidence of adverse effects should be used (the *BNF* cites ibuprofen and diclofenac). After prescribing, the clinician must actively seek the known ill effects. Omeprazole, the gastric acid suppressant, reduces the risk of NSAID-induced gastric bleeding, but does not protect against the other serious side-effects.

Non-drug management of OA

The following are at the centre of functional maintenance and minimizing disability in OA.

- regular physiotherapy to maintain joint mobility and muscular strength
- regular (daily) exercise within the patient's limits. Swimming is particularly good, as it is non-weight-bearing
- weight loss if the patient is obese, to reduce weight-bearing stress on the hips and knees
- in more advanced OA, appliances such as walking aids, joint supports and modifications to home and car.

Clearly the services of the physiotherapist, occupational therapist and dietitian are necessary for these interventions to succeed.

Joint replacement

Few operations can so greatly relieve pain and stiffness, and restore quality of life, as total hip replacement (THR), even in the very elderly. Knee and elbow replacement are well established and shoulder and ankle replacement will soon become so. The operative and post-operative risks are acceptable to most patients (although no one believes 'it will happen to me'!). The joint prostheses have a remarkably long life, dependent on the amount of use they get – they can sometimes be 'revised' (replaced). So the outlook for most OA sufferers is usually positive.

Rheumatoid arthritis (RA)

Both at its onset and over the long term, RA must be managed by a rheumatologist. Only that (and later, shared care) will avoid rapid joint destruction and lifelong pain and disability. However, the following is a brief introduction to the principal features of RA, its diagnosis and management, because the early diagnosis of RA will usually be made (or missed) in primary care.

What is RA?

The cause of RA remains unknown, but autoimmunity (the body's immune mechanisms turning against its own tissues) is involved. Whereas OA is limited to the joint or joints, RA is a systemic process which may involve many other tissues and organs. It affects 1–2% of the population, is more common in women than in men (ratio *c.* 3:1), and its onset is usually earlier than that of OA (20–40 years of age). Two key features of RA must be clearly understood.

1 Joint damage (erosion of cartilage and bone) begins within a few months of the onset of RA. Later, ligaments and tendons may be eroded.

2 Remission of RA occurs in fewer than 20% of patients and rarely lasts as long as a year. In most patients, the disease process continues and the treatment regimen must also continue.

Symptoms and signs of RA

Symptoms

Patients often present with vague malaise, joint aches and stiffness. On questioning, they may admit to unexplained weight loss and will tell you that the joint stiffness persists for one or more hours in the morning, subsiding later in the day. These rather vague early symptoms should set alarm bells ringing for the clinician.

Signs

- On examination, look for symmetrical swelling of the small joints of the hands and/or wrists. The feet (particularly the metatarso-phalangeal joints) may also be affected.
- The swollen joints are usually tender on compression.
- They may be slightly flexed, and straightening them may be uncomfortable.

You should immediately suspect early RA and request the following blood tests:

1 rheumatoid factor

2 erythrocyte sedimentation rate (ESR) > 30 mm/hour

3 an autoimmune antibody screen, which needs expert interpretation.

Refer the patient as 'urgent – 1 month' to a rheumatologist.

Specialist treatment of RA, including shared care

The rheumatologist will confirm the diagnosis using further serology (blood tests), and is then likely to prescribe:

1 an NSAID (see under OA). RA is an inflammatory condition and NSAIDs relieve both pain and inflammation. Unfortunately, despite this, NSAIDs do not arrest the process of joint erosion, and their extensive adverse effects have been outlined in the OA section above

2 a disease-modifying anti-rheumatic drug (DMARD). DMARDs are started once the diagnosis is certain and the severity has been assessed. These drugs not only relieve the symptoms of RA, but they also suppress the disease process gradually over a 6-month period. DMARDs usually reduce the need for NSAIDs, which is very desirable. They have important side-effects (see *BNF*, Chapter 10.1.3), but are less risky than the NSAIDs.

Typically the rheumatologist will start the patient on methotrexate 7.5 mg **weekly**, orally, and build up the dose gradually to a maintenance level of 10 mg to 25 mg **once a week**. A popular alternative is sulfasalazine, 500 mg daily, increasing to 1 gram twice daily by stages.

Methotrexate is an anti-metabolite which interrupts cell division, and it has been used for decades to treat a variety of cancers. It is potentially toxic, even at this low dosage, and the rheumatologist and primary care clinician must actively seek signs of toxicity (see *BNF*, Chapter 10.1.3, including the CSM* advice). Full blood counts and liver function tests must be repeated fortnightly at the start of treatment, then every month once the dose has been stabilized.

Sulfasalazine is a combination of a sulphonamide with a salicylate. It is the sulphonamide moiety which acts as the disease-modifying agent in RA. The sulphonamide element can rarely cause serious blood disorders, and the patient's blood counts (haemoglobin, white cell count and differential white cell count) must be monitored at least monthly for the first 3 months of treatment. Liver function tests must also be done regularly.

Other second-line drugs for RA include leflunomide, hydroxychloroquine, gold injections and d-penicillamine. A group of exciting new biologic agents (etanercept, infliximab and adalimumab) are now available to the rheumatologist. The *BNF* gives brief details of all of these, including their arrays of serious adverse effects. No single anti-rheumatic drug is invariably successful, and several drugs or drug combinations may need to be tried in order to achieve adequate control. The important message is that ongoing joint inflammation will inevitably lead to damage, and must be controlled.

Response to DMARD treatment is assessed as a reduction in the ESR or C-reactive protein. If these parameters do not return to normal, the disease must be treated more aggressively.

The use of steroids in RA treatment

The high-potency synthetic oral steroid, prednisolone, is sometimes given in the early management of RA, to reduce joint inflammation while the DMARD is starting to work (this may take weeks or months). Relief of symptoms is quick and dramatic, and patients will often press for its ongoing use. However, its long-term side-effects mean that it should only be used in the short term for acute flare-ups. An alternative to oral steroids is an intramuscular injection of triamcinolone, which may reduce the risk of a major relapse of joint pain and stiffness once the steroid effect wears off.

* CSM = Committee on Safety of Medicines (UK).

The other important use of steroids in RA is the intra-articular injection of a high-potency steroid such as methylprednisolone. This relieves pain and stiffness within a few days, and the beneficial effect often lasts for weeks or even months.

Non-drug measures in RA management

- The patient should be given a realistic understanding of RA and the need for lifelong co-operation with the various specialties involved in their treatment.

- Individual joints should be rested when the disease is active. Using adjustable supports intermittently and night-time splints is often found to be helpful.

- Exercise is important, under a specialist physiotherapist when the RA is active, including:
  - passive movement of all joints
  - hydrotherapy with gentle active exercise when the disease process is improving
  - in remission, daily exercise within the limits of pain-free movement; an occupational therapist can contribute greatly to the patient's quality of life in the quiescent phase of RA
  - weight loss is essential if the patient is obese.

Conclusion

Few diseases require such skilled management and interprofessional liaison as RA. Even that sometimes fails. Remember that RA is a serious, destructive and chronic condition, with remissions and relapses, in which the full co-operation of the patient can greatly improve both outcome and quality of life.

13 Depression

Introduction

When patients visit you complaining of depression, only a proportion will be found to be clinically depressed. Depression is **not** feeling low in mood for a few days – that happens to most people. Depression is **not** worry or stress at work or at home, although this may contribute to true depression. Depression is **not** the normal grief reaction on the death of a loved one, although that too may precipitate depression. Millions of people have been prescribed modern antidepressant drugs for these and other emotional and societal problems, and have gained little benefit and suffered one or more of the 22½ lines of side-effects noted in the *BNF* (Chapter 4.3.3) for the selective serotonin reuptake inhibitor (SSRI) antidepressants. These are not the 'feel-good' pills they were once claimed to be by the media.

Diagnosing depression

The clinician who suspects depression should seek the following symptoms – the presence of at least four indicates clinical depression:

1. low mood, loss of happiness or equanimity lasting 4 weeks
2. mood not improved by pleasant events or relationships
3. loss of enjoyment of everyday life, lasting 4 weeks
4. loss of interest in things and people, lasting 4 weeks

5 sleep disturbance of various types, from insomnia to spending most of the day in bed

6 difficulty in concentrating and making decisions

7 withdrawal from personal relationships

8 'motor retardation' – slowing of thought processes and physical activity.

In the UK, the National Institute for Clinical Excellence (NICE) recommends that clinical depression be classified as 'mild', 'moderate' or 'severe', and suggests two 'screening' questions to give the clinician a preliminary indication of whether the patient is clinically depressed or not.

- Question 1: 'During the last month, have you often felt down, depressed or hopeless?

- Question 2: 'During the last month, have you often found little interest or pleasure in doing things?'

To these we might add: 'Have you been treated for depression before?'

If the answer to both questions is 'No', the patient is probably not clinically depressed. If the answer to either question is 'Yes', you must proceed to do a full Mental State Examination to seek points 1–8 above (you will learn how to do this in a psychiatry course). Depression is a serious illness, causing much suffering and, in its severe form, carrying a substantial risk of suicide. Remember that patients with severe, suicidal depression will usually have gone through the stages of mild and moderate depression, so these early stages must be treated effectively in order to prevent progression.

Deciding whether a particular patient's depression is mild, moderate or severe needs training and experience, but the World Health Organization (WHO) proposed a decision guide in 1992 (*see* Table 13.1). This is an important table, since appropriate management depends on the initial staging.

Table 13.1: The 10th Revision of the International Classification of Diseases (ICD-10) for the Classification of Depression

Key symptoms	Other symptoms
Persistent sadness or low mood	Disturbed sleep, often with early wakening
Loss of interest or pleasure	Poor concentration or indecisiveness
Fatigue or low energy	Low self-confidence
	Poor or increased appetite
	Suicidal thoughts
	Agitation or slowing of movements
	Guilt or self-blame

- Symptoms should be present for at least 2 weeks.
- Less than 4 symptoms = patient not clinically depressed.
- **Mild depression** = 4 symptoms (including 2 key symptoms), considerable difficulty in continuing with ordinary work, domestic or social activities.
- **Moderate depression** = 5–6 symptoms (including at least 2 key symptoms), considerable difficulty in continuing with ordinary work, domestic or social activities.
- **Severe depression** = ≥ 7 symptoms with or without psychotic features (including all 3 key symptoms), considerable distress or agitation, and unlikely to continue with social, work or domestic activities.

Treating depression

Table 13.2, modified from the NICE Guidelines published in 2004, is a useful guide to the management of depression. Most depression is diagnosed in primary care (as is most other illness), and with training and experience, most mild depression is best treated in primary care (Step 2 in Table 13.2).

Table 13.2: A stepped-care approach to the management of depression

Level	Stage of depression	Intervention
Step 1: GP, practice nurse	Recognition	Assessment
Step 2: GP, practice nurse, primary care mental health worker if available	Mild depression	Watchful waiting Guided self-help Computerised cognitive behaviour therapy (CBT) Exercise Brief psychological interventions, if available
Step 3: Shared care* (hospital and primary care) Primary care mental health worker	Moderate or severe depression	Medication Psychological interventions (Combined treatments)
Step 4: Mental health specialist care	Treatment-resistant depression Recurrent depression Atypical depression Psychotic depression	Medication Complex psychological interventions (Combined treatments)
Step 5: Inpatient care, crisis teams	Risk to life Severe self-neglect	Medication Combined treatments ECT

* 'Shared care' is referral to a psychiatrist for an assessment and management plan, with regular review by the GP and community psychiatric nurse.

Source: Adapted from National Institute for Clinical Excellence (2004) *Management of Depression in Primary and Secondary Care.*

Watchful waiting: Most depression will recover spontaneously, given time. So at the first consultation, sympathetic listening, discussion and advice on measures to improve sleep pattern may be all that is needed, with an appointment for review in no more than a week. Regular, rhythmic exercise should be strongly advised, as it has been shown to improve all levels of depression (30 minutes per day of brisk walking, jogging, swimming or cycling, according to the patient's physical ability). Antidepressant drugs should not be prescribed for mild depression, at least for the first month. Sedatives and hypnotics should not be given, as they worsen depression and often lead to habituation.

Cognitive behavioural therapy (CBT) and brief psychotherapy have been proved to be therapeutic in mild and moderate depression. Both aim to readjust the patient's thought processes away from a negative self-image and attitude towards a positive one. Both need training, and trained psychotherapists are often unavailable in primary care. A form of CBT that is delivered by computer has proved useful for some patients, but is not a satisfactory alternative for most.

Unless a member of the primary care team has training and experience in psychiatry, or a specialist community-based team can help, patients who are assessed as moderately to severely depressed should be referred to a psychiatrist on an urgent basis. This ensures the necessary expertise to formulate a management plan, including the most appropriate antidepressant. Thereafter, care can be mainly in general practice, with hospital visits for psychotherapy (or community psychotherapy, if available), occasional review by a psychiatrist, and urgent review/admission if the condition deteriorates and/or if suicidal symptoms occur. That is Step 3.

Severe depression (*see* Table 13.1) requires urgent referral to a psychiatrist for drug treatment and specialist psychological treatment (Step 4). Step 5 is psychiatric inpatient care, where there is a risk of self-harm, harm to others or severe self-neglect. 'Formal' admission is sometimes unavoidable (i.e. legally enforced admission with or without the patient's consent).

Drug treatment of depression

This will be described in outline only, since selection of the most appropriate drug and its combination with psychotherapy and lifestyle measures requires specialist training, to which this can serve only as a brief introduction. Chapters 10 and 17 of *How Drugs Work* give an outline of the pharmacology (science) of these drugs, so far as it is known. They should be read (or re-read) before proceeding.

The billion neurons (nerve cells) in the central nervous system (CNS) communicate with each other and with other parts of the brain and body by means of chemical signals – the neurotransmitters (see *How Drugs Work*, Chapter 10). It is probable that in moderate and severe depression, this normal neuronal communication is disrupted. Since the two main types of antidepressant drugs are known (in animal tissue experiments) to increase the availability of one or more neurotransmitters at nerve endings in the CNS, it was postulated in 1965 that depression might be associated with reduced neurotransmission due to reduced production of chemical signals or their accelerated breakdown (see *How Drugs Work*, Chapter 17). It may be decades before the neurochemical disorders of depression are understood. In the meantime, all of the drugs listed below cure or improve a majority of depressed patients, which was not possible before their discovery.

At the outset, the following should be emphasized.

- Patients should never be prescribed a combination of two antidepressants in primary care (this requires a specialist decision and supervision, and can be dangerous).

- Most of the antidepressants that are licensed for use in primary care take 4–8 weeks to relieve the depression, in most patients. This must be clearly explained to the patient (and carer) in order to avoid disappointment resulting in non-compliance. Review the patient every 1–2 weeks until improvement occurs.

- Once the depression has 'lifted', **the antidepressant must be continued at the same dose for at least 6 months.** This prolonged treatment greatly increases the likelihood of a prolonged remission (and sometimes a permanent cure). A short course of treatment incurs a greater risk of rapid relapse.

- When the treatment course is complete, the antidepressant should be withdrawn gradually, reducing the dose over 4 weeks to avoid the many unpleasant side-effects of withdrawal (see *BNF*, Chapter 4.3, monograph).

- If there has been no improvement in the symptoms within 8 weeks:
  - consider the possibility of non-compliance or erratic compliance – both are common with antidepressants, due to their side-effects (listed in the *BNF*). If compliance appears satisfactory:
  - try to obtain psychotherapy (this is often difficult), and encourage the

patient to take regular exercise; both of these improve the response to drug treatment

- increase the dose of the original drug, and if there has still been no response within a further 4 weeks
- refer the patient to a psychiatrist as a matter of urgency.

The main antidepressant drug groups

These are, in order of frequency of prescribing:

1 the selective serotonin reuptake inhibitors (SSRIs)

2 the tricyclic antidepressants (TCAs) and related drugs

3 other antidepressants (a *BNF* 'classification')

4 the monoamine-oxidase inhibitors (MAOIs) and the single reversible inhibitor of monoamine oxidase (RIMA, a more recent drug). **These are for specialist use only** (or shared care).

The individual drugs in all of these groups act so as to increase the 'availability' in the CNS of the monoamine neurotransmitters noradrenaline, serotonin (5-hydroxytryptamine) and/or dopamine. Some are more specific ('selective') for one monoamine than the others, although 'selectivity' is relative (see *How Drugs Work*, Chapter 6). Because of this, different drugs have different side-effects, and their side-effect profile may determine their choice for a particular patient. For example, an anxious depressed patient (agitated depression) may benefit from the sedative side-effect of a TCA, e.g. amitriptyline, nortriptyline or lofepramine. Conversely, a lethargic patient may be prescribed an SSRI, most of which have an alerting side-effect. However, in non-lethargic patients, SSRIs can cause a degree of agitation in the first 2 weeks of treatment.

Selection of the most appropriate antidepressant must take into account the following factors in particular:

1 **suicide risk** – the TCAs are cardiotoxic in overdose, and the SSRIs in normal doses may cause suicidal thoughts in patients who were not initially suicidal

2 **existing chronic disease** – the TCAs should be used with great caution in the elderly and in patients with cardiac disease, epilepsy, glaucoma,

urinary retention and other conditions (see *BNF*, Chapter 4.3.1, amitriptyline and Chapter 4.3.3, SSRI introduction). The SSRIs require caution in patients with epilepsy, cardiac disease, diabetes, glaucoma and bleeding disorders. Both groups require caution in patients with impaired liver function

3 **existing drug treatment** – the *BNF* (Appendix 1, 'Antidepressants') lists the many drug–drug interactions of the antidepressants

4 **previously successful antidepressant treatment** – should usually be considered first choice.

Points 1 to 3 above should warn the beginner of the problems and dangers of antidepressant treatment. They also show how desirable it is to avoid drug treatment in mild depression. Observe your teaching psychiatrists at work, and question them about their drug selection rationale.

Two other depressive diagnoses

Dysthymia

Dysthymic patients have persistently depressed mood, on most days, for most of the day, sometimes lasting for years. They cannot be diagnosed as 'depressed' under criteria 1 to 8 at the start of this chapter, because their symptoms are less severe and rather different:

- feeling 'bleak and hopeless'
- poor concentration
- fatigue – 'tired all the time' (TATT)
- insomnia or hypersomnia
- anorexia or overeating.

It is very important to recognise and diagnose dysthymia, for it can blight a person's life and that of their family, and may last a decade, if untreated. Furthermore, it usually responds to antidepressant drug treatment (with a TCA or SSRI), but does not respond well to psychotherapy. It rarely requires specialist intervention. One in 30 people will develop dysthymia at some time.

Manic-depressive disorder (bipolar illness)

This is a psychotic illness characterized by episodic mood swings from extreme elation, hyperactivity, irritability and socially disruptive behaviour to severe depression. It is far removed from the relatively small mood swings that are experienced by many (perhaps most) normal people.

Manic-depressive disorder requires specialist management. Lithium carbonate is usually effective in 'ironing out' the peaks and troughs of mood, but it is a dangerous drug whose therapeutic dose is close to its toxic dose. Most psychiatric units have a special 'lithium outpatient clinic', where patients come monthly to have their serum lithium concentration checked and their progress assessed. Attempts are made to trace defaulters, as lithium toxicity is life-threatening (see *How Drugs Work*, Chapter 17) and it is a drug-related psychiatric emergency, requiring immediate Accident and Emergency admission.

Specialists are now using the anti-epileptic valproic acid or antipsychotics such as olanzapine, together with lithium, in the acute phase of a manic attack. These drugs control the condition rapidly, whereas lithium requires several days to exert its anti-manic effect (see *BNF*, Chapter 4.2.3).

The serotonergic syndrome

This is described briefly because, although uncommon, its early recognition will be missed if the doctor or nurse is unaware of it. It is a life-threatening emergency, usually occurring in an elderly patient on a high SSRI dosage or an SSRI combined with an MAOI (which includes the anti-parkinsonian drugs selegiline and rasagiline). If such a patient becomes agitated or confused, look for shivering, tremor, increased reflexes and increased temperature. Admit the patient to Accident and Emergency as an emergency, **stating your diagnosis.**

Electroconvulsive therapy (ECT)

In ECT, an electric shock applied across the patient's temples causes a generalized CNS convulsion. It relieves up to 85% of severe depression in cases where combined treatment has failed, or on initial hospital admission, where the risk to the patient precludes drug treatment, with its prolonged delay in response. ECT is without credible rationale, but it works!

14 Anxiety and agitation

Introduction

Anxiety is commonplace in human life. It is the mental and physical response to perceived threats, stressors and dreads ranging from physical dangers to workplace problems, worries about loved ones, financial problems and many others. Humans are generally very good at coping with these stressors. Close-knit agrarian communities, tribes and clans have in the past given the individual invaluable support in managing their anxiety. Inevitably, modern industrialized society has largely lost these social supporting practices, and people whose inbuilt coping mechanisms are inadequate, or whose stressors are too great, often turn for help to doctors and nurses in primary care. More than one stressor is often present, and a family history of anxiety predisposes the individual to an anxiety disorder, as does learned behaviour, such as growing up in a tense and nervous environment. If the focus of a patient's apprehensive expectation is *multiple life* circumstances, then they are diagnosed as having 'generalized anxiety disorder.'

The problem of managing anxiety in primary care

Unfortunately, doctors and nurses in NHS primary care may not have enough time or skill to provide adequate non-drug support, and community psychotherapists are in short supply. Sedative/anxiolytic drugs are initially very effective in relieving the symptoms of anxiety, but they all rapidly cease to have any effect. The patient needs increasing doses, leading to chronic sedative dependence, in which a patient continues to take high doses of the sedative or hypnotic to avoid the withdrawal effects of stopping, and with no anxiolytic benefit whatever. It is therefore a reflection upon both clinicians and modern society that almost 10% of the western population are taking sedatives or hypnotics. In the same context, the current epidemic of substance abuse and addiction may cause people to present with symptoms of anxiety that are actually symptoms of withdrawal. This should be kept in mind.

Anxiety involves the body as well as the mind

The individual's response to stress is dependent on their personality, physiology and life experience. Humankind has inherited the primitive 'fight or flight' response to anxiety – the mammalian physiological response necessary for survival in nature. This includes the secretion of the 'stress hormones' – adrenaline and cortisol – by the adrenal glands. These have profound effects on the heart, arteries, muscles, lungs and intestines, causing somatic (physical) symptoms (see below). Most of these are of no value in modern society, but increase the patient's distress. Adrenaline also feeds back to the central nervous system (CNS), worsening the psychological symptoms of anxiety.

Diagnosing generalized anxiety disorder

Look for both the psychological and the somatic symptoms, for the extent of both allows you to assess the severity of the anxiety. Don't forget that a patient may present with only one or two symptoms – you must actively seek the 'full picture' as follows.

Psychological symptoms

Present on most days for at least a month:

* fear, dread
* worry which cannot be 'switched off'
* irritability

- poor concentration
- insomnia, particularly difficulty in getting to sleep. (*Early wakening is more common in depression.*)

Somatic (physical) symptoms

- 'My heart is beating faster' – tachycardia
- Nausea, stomach pains/cramps, heartburn
- Fine tremor of hands

Somatic signs

On physical examination, you may find:

- tachycardia (rapid heart rate)
- hypertension (raised blood pressure)
- fine tremor of outstretched hands
- hyper-reflexia
- dilated pupils.

Treatment of generalized anxiety

Initially, the benzodiazepine hypnotics and anxiolytics give immediate, very effective relief of anxiety (see *How Drugs Work*, Chapter 12, for their mode of action). Tables 14.1 and 14.2 are reproduced from that chapter, and summarize the known characteristics of these drugs. There is much overlap – the hypnotics cause some daytime sedation and the sedatives (anxiolytics) promote sleep at night. As explained in the introduction above, their effect wears off within as little as a week, after which their use should be intermittent, or you will have produced a benzodiazepine-dependent patient. Beta-adrenergic blockers such as propranolol will improve the somatic symptoms but do nothing for the psychological symptoms (see *BNF*, Chapter 2.4). That leaves us with a major problem – what to do next – for the anxiety is unlikely to have gone away.

Table 14.1: Anxiolytics/sedatives

Name	Half-life (hours)	Approved uses according to the British National Formulary (BNF)
Benzodiazepine anxiolytics		
diazepam	20–40	*Oral:* Short-term relief of severe anxiety. Must never be used alone in depression or agitated depression (suicide risk). Causes drowsiness, giddiness and staggering (ataxia), and confusion, especially in the elderly. For other side effects, see *BNF* *Intravenous:* Status epilepticus, panic attacks, acute alcohol withdrawal. Always use the emulsion (Diazemuls) *Rectal:* Where the oral or intravenous route is unavailable (absorption is rapid) Benzodiazepines are of no value in preventing epilepsy
lorazepam oxazepam	8–12	*Oral:* Short-term relief of severe anxiety. Similar side-effects to diazepam. Useful in patients with impaired liver function *Intravenous:* IV lorazepam is now the preferred treatment of status epilepticus
Non-benzodiazepine anxiolytics		
buspirone		Short-term relief of anxiety, but takes up to 2 weeks to act. Best used with specialist consultation. Inhibits serotonin ($5HT_{1A}$) receptors and some CNS noradrenaline receptors
beta-blockers		Reduce tremor and palpitations but have no effect on worry, tension or fear. For details of action, see *How Drugs Work*, Chapter 6. Tense snooker players have found them helpful because of the physical effect of reducing tremor!

Table 14.2 Hypnotics/sleep-inducing drugs

Name	Half-life (hours)	Approved uses according to the British National Formulary (BNF)
Benzodiazepine hypnotics		
loprazolam lormetazepam temazepam	8–12	Short-term use (1 week) as hypnotics and anxiolytics. Cause a few hangover effects. Withdrawal effects common if use is prolonged
nitrazepam flurazepam flunitrazepam	16–30	Short-term use (1 week). All cause drowsiness and giddiness next day, with amnesia. Cause confusion and staggering (ataxia) in the elderly. Dependence develops rapidly. Avoid flunitrazepam, which is particularly liable to abuse
diazepam	20–40	Occasionally useful as a single dose at night, where the insomnia is associated with daytime anxiety. Sedation continues well into the next day, due to the long-acting metabolite nordiazepam
Non-benzodiazepine hypnotics		
zaleplon zolpidem zopiclone	1 2 4	These have few advantages over the benzodiazepines. They act on the same $GABA_A$ receptors. For short-term use only. They have many more side-effects than the benzodiazepines.
clomethiazole	5	Occasionally useful in elderly patients but not routinely. Relatively free from hangover effects. Dangerous interaction with alcohol

The mainstays of anxiety management are not drugs. They are:

1 the supportive practitioner–patient relationship

2 psychological treatment, if available

3 behavioural therapy

4 social therapy.

This is a complex territory, but often curative, and every clinician should be able to offer the patient at least one of these.

Practitioner–patient relationship

- Accept the distress.
- Seek to relate the anxiety to one or more adverse events – everyone will 'crack' if stressed enough. Arrange regular weekly or fortnightly appointments with the same practitioner.
- Adopt a realistic but optimistic attitude.
- 'Ride along' with the ups and downs in progress.
- Refer the patient to a specialist if necessary.

Psychological treatment

- Devise and agree appropriate lifestyle changes so as to eliminate or reduce the stressors.
- Arrange group therapy – sharing experiences with others having the same problem – if available.
- Refer more serious patients for the much more advanced psychotherapy available to a psychiatrist.

Behavioural therapy

This usually involves 'biofeedback', in which the patient is taught techniques for decreasing the various symptoms. It needs a specialist or a clinician with special training, and is a good example of the advantages of clinicians with special skills/interest in primary care.

Social therapy

This should include a three-pronged programme to improve the patient's environment.

1 Include the family members or 'significant others' in therapy – understanding the problems and how to behave so as to support the patient.
2 Seek 'peer support' – encouraging the patient's friends to accept and live with the problems. This is often difficult.
3 Involve the patient's employer, if this is feasible, to remove excessive work

stressors, including the fear of dismissal. A doctor's or nurse's communication can make the difference between 'the sack' and the retention of a valuable employee.

Conclusion

Remember that this is a very brief introduction to a complex socio-medical problem, involving a holistic approach more than drug treatment. The more complex anxiety disorders – panic disorder, obsessive-compulsive disorder, phobic disorder and dissociative disorder – are beyond the scope of this introductory text.

15 Important adverse drug reactions and drug:drug interactions

A number of drugs in common clinical practice are likely to cause problems (*see* Table 15.1). Some are naturally very toxic, others become toxic when liver or kidney function is impaired, while some interact with a large selection of other drugs. Severe allergic reactions can also occur with a number of compounds.

Types of adverse reaction

Adverse drug reactions account for about 2% of acute hospital admissions and occur in 10–20% of hospital inpatients. Type A reactions are those which can be predicted from the known action of the drug, whereas Type B reactions are unpredictable and unrelated to the dose administered. There are two main causes of type A reactions – decreased removal by the liver and kidney and excessive sensitivity to the action of the drug. For example, the slow metabolism (breaking down) of morphine by the liver in patients with liver damage can cause excessive sedation and even coma. Impaired elimination of digoxin by the kidney can result in anorexia, nausea, heart irregularities and disturbance of colour vision. Increased sensitivity to the action of digoxin can also occur in patients with a low potassium concentration in the blood, and patients with chest disease are more susceptible to the depressant effect of morphine on respiration.

Type B reactions are unusual and unexpected. There are a number of factors which make the patient more likely to develop these adverse effects. Certain enzymes (chemicals which convert one substance to another) are

Table 15.1: Examples of drugs which commonly cause problems

Type 1	Adverse effect	Type 2	Adverse effect
amiodarone	Thyroid abnormalities	amiodarone	Photosensitivity
corticosteroids	Osteoporosis Cataracts Infections	flucloxacillin co-amoxiclav	Jaundice
digoxin	Anorexia Heart rhythm disturbance	antimalarials	Haemolysis
diuretics	Electrolyte abnormalities	oral contraceptives	Jaundice
insulin	Hypoglycaemia	antithyroid drugs	Bone-marrow suppression
non-steroidal anti-inflammatory agents	Gastrointestinal bleeding	aspirin	Rashes Hypersensitivity reactions
theophylline	Heart rhythm disturbance Vomiting Epileptic seizures	penicillins	Rashes Anaphylaxis
warfarin	Bleeding	warfarin	Rashes Hypersensitivity reactions

absent from red blood cells of Afro-Caribbeans, making them more susceptible to haemolysis (breakdown of red cells) when a number of drugs (e.g. antimalarials, painkillers, antimicrobials) are administered. Environmental factors – diet, pollution, intake of alcohol, tobacco and other recreational drugs – are also probably important, but these have not been studied in sufficient detail to allow accurate predictions. Allergic reactions are very important, and have been studied in more detail. These types of reaction mean that the patient has been previously exposed to the drug, although they may not always be aware of this. The exposure results in the formation of an antibody against the drug. Antibodies are proteins which are formed in the body in response to a foreign material (an antigen). In clinical practice, antibiotics (especially penicillins) are the most likely cause. The antibody becomes attached to the surface of certain cells called mast cells. The mast cells are destroyed, releasing a number of substances such as histamine and prostaglandins which make blood vessels dilate and so reduce the blood pressure. This can result in allergic rashes, but the most severe reaction is anaphylaxis. The onset of this condition is rapid, with chest pain, pallor, collapse, wheeze and low blood pressure. Immediate treatment with intra-muscular adrenaline is essential. Other examples of allergic reactions include haemolysis (antibodies attached to red cells causing them to break down), depression of the bone marrow, jaundice and kidney damage.

Adverse reactions cannot be eliminated altogether, but they can be minimized by taking a drug history from every patient for previous adverse effects, reducing the number of drugs if possible, and remembering that certain individuals are more likely to experience adverse effects, e.g. the elderly and those with liver or kidney disease. Always bear in mind that an unexpected change in a patient's condition may be due to an adverse drug reaction.

Drug interactions

We have now reached the era of evidence-based polypharmacy. A patient with diabetes and associated cardiovascular disease is likely to be taking more than 10 drugs, all of proven efficacy. The greater the number of drugs that a patient receives, the greater the risk of drug interactions. Dangerous interactions are also likely in seriously ill hospitalized patients, in the elderly, and when drugs with a small difference between the therapeutic and toxic dose are used.

As with adverse effects, most interactions occur with drugs at their site of action or because the routes of elimination are affected. Serious interactions have also been described when different drugs are mixed for intravenous administration. The addition of sodium bicarbonate can cause a drug to come out of solution and remain suspended in the liquid, e.g. diazepam and some anti cancer drugs. Drugs should never be added to blood, as important interactions are likely to occur with a number of blood elements.

Interactions at the site of action

In a recent large study in north-west England, involving almost 20,000 patients admitted to hospital, this was by far the most important type of interaction. The commonest adverse effect was bleeding due to aspirin, and the risk was increased by co-administration of anti-inflammatory agents (NSAIDs), antiplatelet drugs and warfarin. Interactions at the site of action can be additive or antagonistic. The combination of diazepam and alcohol producing excessive sedation is an example of an additive effect, and combinations of antihypertensive drugs can cause excessive reductions in blood pressure. An important antagonist effect is observed when beta-blockers such as atenolol are combined with beta-agonists such as salbutamol. The bronchodilator effect of salbutamol is reduced and the effect of the beta-blocker on heart rate is impaired.

Interactions at the site of elimination

Several drugs are broken down in the liver, where enzymes can be altered in two important ways. The enzymes can become more active, so that other drugs are broken down more rapidly and their effect is diminished (enzyme induction). Rifampicin, a drug that is widely used to treat tuberculosis, and drugs used to treat epilepsy are good examples of enzyme inducers. Warfarin is the most important drug to be affected in this way. Enzyme inducers will decrease the effect of warfarin so that the patient's blood is more likely to clot. Doctors will increase the dose of warfarin to overcome the reduced effect. The patient will then be at no increased risk unless the enzyme inducer is stopped. If this occurs, the patient is now more likely to bleed. Drugs that suppress enzyme activity are even more dangerous, because their effect is rapid. Cimetidine, an ulcer-healing drug and enzyme inhibitor, if given to a patient on warfarin will prevent the breakdown of warfarin and increase the risk of bleeding over a very short time period.

Competition for removal by the kidney can also occur. Thiazide diuretics block the renal excretion of lithium, a drug used to treat bipolar disease, and increase the risk of lithium toxicity.

Clinical importance of drug interactions

Most documented drug interactions are of little clinical significance. Interactions become important when the dose of a drug is critical and a small change in the amount of drug in the body results in toxicity or lack of therapeutic effect. It is impossible to remember all possible drug interactions, but be on the alert when certain drugs are being administered (*see* Table 15.2).

Table 15.2: Drugs commonly involved in important interactions

ACE inhibitors	diuretics
anti-epileptic drugs	hypoglycaemic agents (antidiabetics)
antidepressants	lithium
anti-inflammatory drugs	oral contraceptives
amiodarone	rifampicin
beta-blockers	theophylline
cimetidine	warfarin
digoxin	

Many patients do not regard alcohol as a drug, but it can interact with a number of prescription drugs, including the following:

- metronidazole – interferes with the metabolism of alcohol, causing flushing, headache, sweating and nausea

- hypnotics and sedatives – sedative effect is potentiated

- warfarin – increased anticoagulant effect after acute administration; reduced effect after chronic administration.

Remember also that the interacting agent may be an 'over-the-counter' drug. The combination of aspirin with an anti-inflammatory drug is the commonest cause of bleeding from the stomach. *How Drugs Work* (2e), Chapters 23 and 24 contain further information on this important topic. Preventable prescription-related illness is a major cause of hospitalization and death.

16 Some thoughts on infectious diseases

These are among the commonest diseases. There are hundreds of infectious diseases involving every organ in the body, and often the entire body. Many are minor and self-limiting (recovery occurs within a few days without intervention), many are severe enough to need nursing and medical support, and many are often fatal. AIDS, pneumonia, enteritis, malaria, tuberculosis and measles remain the commonest causes of child death in developing countries. This subject requires a large textbook even for an introduction, and apart from the chapter on the treatment of community-acquired pneumonia, no other infectious diseases have been considered in this short book.

However, a few principles may be helpful by way of a realistic orientation with regard to this large topic, which is likely to become increasingly important over the coming decades, as current antimicrobial drugs become ineffective.

The body is not defenceless!

For millions of years before modern medicine, the human body has been invaded by a wide range of other living organisms – micro-organisms (such as viruses, bacteria and yeasts), single-celled protozoans (such as malaria), and a variety of larger parasites which invade the skin, intestine, liver, lung, muscle and brain. The powerful human immune system produces specific antibodies which circulate in the bloodstream and, working together with cell-mediated immunity, destroy viruses, bacteria and yeasts wherever they have lodged, ensuring recovery in the majority of cases. Following the infection, 'memory cells' in the immune system carry a residual immunity for each specific infection, and this often lasts for years. Modern vaccination schedules (see *BNF*, Chapter 14.1) ensure that, by the age of 5 years, the majority of western populations have high levels of immunity to the most dangerous, life-threatening infections such as diphtheria, tetanus and polio-myelitis, and to infections that seldom kill but which can have serious sequelae (after-effects) in a minority of patients, such as mumps, measles and whooping-cough.

Virus infections

These range from the common cold and 'flu to the childhood fevers such as measles, mumps, German measles, chickenpox and glandular fever (adolescents), to the viruses that cause aseptic meningitis, hepatitis, rabies and encephalitis, and the modern international scourge of retroviruses causing human immune deficiency (AIDS). Yet other viruses have been implicated in the aetiology (causation) of cancers, e.g. hepatitis B and C viruses in liver cancer, papillomavirus in cervical cancer in young women, and HTL virus in leukaemia.

The treatment of most viral infections is symptomatic and involves managing complications. Several 'families' of antiviral drugs are available, e.g. the many anti-retrovirals for AIDS (all with serious adverse effects), acyclovir for viral ulceration of the eye (dendritic ulcer) and lamivudine for chronic hepatitis B. Viruses develop resistance to all of these, and most strains of HIV/AIDS require three antiviral drugs to achieve control, despite the toxicity of these drugs. Drug toxicity is often acceptable when no treatment means suffering and death.

The mainstay of management of viral illnesses is vaccination, wherever that is possible. A number of cancers are associated with virus infections, and early vaccination greatly reduces the risk of developing the cancer later in life, e.g. vaccination against the human papilloma virus is now available to protect prepubescent girls from cervical cancer.

Treating bacterial infections

From about 1935, clinicians have had at their disposal an increasing range of antibacterial drugs capable of killing invading bacteria, usually without great risk to the patient. Starting with the sulfonamides, and then the penicillins, the anti-tuberculous drugs, the tetracyclines, the cephalosporins, the macrolides and the 4-quinolones, every decade has seen the discovery of a new family of effective and relatively safe drugs. In the 1960s, it was thought that death from bacterial infections was a thing of the past. In *How Drugs Work*, Chapter 22 gives a concise description of the antibacterial actions of these drugs. It also describes how bacteria develop resistance to them, for the overuse of antibacterial drugs in medicine, veterinary medicine and farming has driven the development and natural selection of resistant strains of all pathogenic (disease-causing) bacteria.

Worse still, resistant bacteria can share their resistance genes with other bacteria of their own and different species, so that resistance to several antibacterials (multi-drug resistance) is now common. And it is not only hospital 'bugs' like MRSA and *Clostridium difficile* which leave clinicians as impotent as with most viral infections, but bacteria in the community, causing pneumonia, stomach ulcers, TB, gonorrhoea and others, which are showing multi-drug resistance in the community.

Patients infected by such resistant organisms will gain no benefit from commonly used antibacterial drugs, and will rely entirely on their own immune mechanisms, as they did before the antibacterial era. Most will recover, but a proportion will die, and some who recover will have permanent organ damage. Several thousand people die every year as a result of resistant infections in UK hospitals, and this pattern is likely to become common in primary care over the coming decades.

Furthermore, due to the effect of antibacterial drugs in unbalancing the delicate symbiosis of the body's extensive flora of bacteria (the skin, mucous membranes, nose, throat and colon have large populations of bacteria which cause no problems and deny access to the tissues by pathogenic bacteria), serious antibacterial-associated diseases such as *Clostridium difficile* colitis kill hundreds of patients per year, as do the allergic reactions of some patients to antibiotics (anaphylactic shock).

For all of these reasons, we recommend that you read and note the 6-monthly *BNF* guidance on antibacterial choice for the main bacterial infections that are common in the community (see *BNF*, Chapter 5.1, Table 1). This incorporates current knowledge of antibacterial resistance of the pathogen which most commonly causes each infection. Your microbiology laboratory should be able to give you regular updates on the main bacterial sensitivities in your community or hospital, to guide your prescribing further.

Antibacterial prescribing should be a science, not a gamble!

Although you will soon discover that it is common practice, the 'blind prescribing' of antibacterial drugs (without proof of the pathogen) is to be deplored, except in life-threatening infectious emergencies such as meningococcal septicaemia and community-acquired pneumonia (CAP – *see* Chapter 9). Appropriate samples (e.g. 'swabs') should always be taken before treatment, and sent for bacteriological culture and sensitivity to different antibacterial agents. This usually takes 24–48 hours, and antibacterial treatment need not be given before that unless there is evidence of systemic spread of the infection. There are three reasons for sending specimens to the laboratory:

1 to identify the pathogen

2 to determine which antibacterial drugs will kill it

3 to enable the laboratory to build up an epidemiological profile of bacterial resistance in its catchment area.

Failure to follow this best practice has led to gross over-prescribing of antibacterial drugs for upper respiratory infections in particular. Around 70% of these are viral in origin, and antibacterial drugs confer no benefit whatsoever, and expose the patient to the risks of antibacterial drugs. As in all your treatment of common disease, try as far as possible to be a clinical scientist!

Index